Practical Application Of Forensic Dentistry

Heath C. Winkler, D.D.S.

Introduction

The search for truth through the use of scientific methodology in forensic sciences has been popularized for decades by various media. We are intuitively prompted by actual cases or realistic fiction to apply logic and reasoning, the core principles of forensic science, to discover truth. There are many aspects of forensics. Accounting, law, pathology, cyber and dentistry are a few examples. This book is written for a newcomer to Forensic Dentistry and will expose the reader to what a Forensic Dentist would experience in his or her field. A young reader who has not decided on a career path will find it useful as a reference. The contents of the pages are not saturated with scientific terminology and take on a conversational tone designed to educate the reader and expose him or her to what a Forensic Dentist strives to accomplish when involved in a forensic identification case of a decedent. Covered are a variety of postmortem identification cases the forensic dentist might experience when presented with the different conditions of the decedents. The goal of the book is to make the reader feel he or she is standing next to the forensic dentist from the time of the notification of a case is received until the identification is complete. The reader is the new assistant who gets exposure to other professionals, several different postmortem conditions, equipment, techniques, scientific methodology, manners, and interpretation and conclusion protocols. Conveyance of findings and what one signs one's name to is exceedingly important and will be covered. The topics of manners, respect and humility will be reviewed although these may seem inconsequential to forensic science and methodology. To illustrate: people involved with science for decades, have spent very little time, if any, on addressing the concept of working well with others. There are two sides to the Forensic Dentistry process. Number one: the Forensic Dentist deals with a decedent who was discovered in less than ideal circumstances and conditions. Brutal homicides, decomposition, fires etc. take the lives of many that become forensic cases [decedents]. They were living breathing members of society that often experienced a painful horrific end of life. It is best to consider yourself fortunate you or a loved one is not on the table. Everyone, including yourself, will benefit from you being respectful of the situation, the people you interact with on the case, and the decedent. Number two: as a Forensic Dentist you're also going to interact with many different professionals from the start of an identification dental case to its conclusion. Every member of this chain deals with death and often the dark side of human existence. The forensic dentist is important but is only a single link in the forensic chain and the planets do not rotate just around him or her. Be confident and lead by example and at the same time present yourself as courteous, humble, friendly, and helpful. Manners cost nothing and can have an exponentially large payoff for you and fellow forensic professionals. Listening is a lost art that is worth its weight in gold. With your phone off, make eye contact with the person talking to you. Listen carefully and you will learn volumes. This skill set in this age of distracting forces requires a little bit of your time and patience. It takes discipline and concentration not to dismiss the person's thoughts or to go to "one upmanship." Leave your ego at the door and start with a blank slate. Mastering good listening skills will win you wonderful forensic allies and make the entire process of dental identification easier and more rewarding for all concerned. The last two paragraphs may seem like basic kindergarten concepts, but I really feel they are as important as any other information in this book and taking them to heart makes you and everyone around you better at their jobs and lives.

I hope you enjoy the book and leave with a better understanding of how Forensic Dentistry and its interactions with other disciplines is applied to each case of a decedent's identification.

Table of Contents

Chapter 1

Chapter I.
Forensic Investigation

Law Enforcement is typically called to the location of a decedent. There they assess the situation. They make sure the scene is clear of danger. The area is blocked off from foot traffic and any other contamination. Notes, photographs, and measurements are taken. The decedent is evaluated, and it is determined their life has ended. When these tasks are completed, Forensic Investigators are called in to take the next steps in processing the scene and gathering information.

Forensic Investigators need to be aware of many things. A few examples are how temperatures effect a decedent and how insect and animal activity effect a decedent. Rigor mortis, liver mortis, and mummification are only a few of the conditions a human can be found in. Forensic Investigators have to know how to properly collect the decedent and surrounding evidence without contaminating or damaging anything that will be used for identification and the deliverance of justice and closure.

Forensic Investigators also need to determine if foul play is suspected. Death by natural occurrences is handled by a different sequence of investigation than a homicide. Properly evaluating the situation will lead to family members getting answers to a terrible situation with their loved ones. This will eventually lead to identification, what occurred, who was involved, justice, closure, and healing. If there is foul play involved, proper evidence collection, and meticulous, regimented information gathering can help provide the victim and their family the justice they deserve.

The Forensic Investigators comb through the scene. They take notes. They photograph the decedent and the surrounding area. They examine the decedent and collect and label anything found on or around the decedent that may be pertinent to explaining the cause of death. They are careful to label collected evidence and record proper chain of custody so there are no questions to the validity of the evidence.

The Forensic Investigator then collects the body to be taken to the morgue. With the assistance of other Forensic technicians, they draw blood samples and take fingerprints if possible. They then take radiographs, weigh, and photograph the decedent. They also package clothes and belongings and document the process.

If there was an automobile involved in the death of a person or people, the entire vehicle may be brought to the morgue and be torn apart meticulously for evidence collection. Investigators can communicate information to the pathologists that may help with the next phase of evidence and information collection. Everything the investigator does effects what the pathologist has to do. Thorough and organized work by the forensic investigator facilitates the pathologist's work.

Forensic Investigators work with Law Enforcement, fire departments, pathologists, victims' families, morticians, hospitals, forensic dentists, and media to bring a decedent's cause of death to public record. Once the cause of death and identification of the decedent is determined, it is often the Forensic Investigator that contacts the victim's family members, media, and law enforcement. Investigators can also contact the funeral director or mortician so the victim can be properly processed for burial services and family's final respects.

Forensic Investigators have an extremely important role in death investigation. They are exposed to some of the darkest acts human beings can inflict upon another person. It can be a stressful profession. Without their expertise and training many questions would go unanswered about what lead up to someone's death and many victims would not receive the justice they deserve. In addition, many of their families would go on, possibly indefinitely, suffering with not knowing what happened to their loved ones.

Forensic Investigators are trained to observe and process information, no matter how seemingly insignificant it is, that could be used to help bring light to an unknown situation regarding a decedent. They are meticulous about recording data and tracking the chain of evidence so everything is accounted for and can be retrieved as needed. They look for natural order and what makes sense and anything out of place catches their eye.

Forensic Investigators that excel in their profession also possess the ability to work well and communicate well with others. They are professionals in a difficult field and deal with the worst situations. They develop a thick skin but at the same time maintain a softness about them. Forensic Investigators have empathy and patience for the family and friends of the victims/decedents even when the anguish they are going through can come out as hostility toward them. They continue to perform their duties in very poor and often dangerous crime scenes where decedents are found. They are exposed to diseases, insects, odors, decay, and hostile individuals. Forensic Investigators push through these adversities toward their goals of cause of death discovery and justice.

I have had the privilege of working with several wonderful investigators over the past 18 years of being a Forensic Dentist. I have learned a lot by following their lead: behavior, attention to detail, professionalism, and ability to deal with awful situations by focusing on specific goals. I have found them to be very helpful and ready to work with me (the Forensic Dentist) at any time. They certainly deserve respect for doing a job that few could accomplish.

In return, when I am called to the morgue to work on a case, I maintain modesty and politeness. I am patient and try to be aware of the amount of stress that is in the room. I don't need to add to it by being bossy, needy, or impatient. I utilize please and thank you. I help set up the equipment I need and help set up the body on the gurney. When I am done, I help wipe and clean everything and take the time to put away the equipment I used. I thank whoever was there for their help and let them know they are appreciated. Amazingly this behavior is most often reciprocated. I think there are enough negatives in a forensic investigator's life, or anyone else's, that someone treating them well is received well.

I find that over time using this approach has led to incredible amounts of politeness and help coming my way from the teams of investigators, techs, and pathologists I work with. For me, it makes the experience much better, and I know I have good people I can count on for help.

Notes Chapter One

Chapter 2

Chapter II.
The Forensic Pathologist

Once the Forensic Investigators and technicians have completed their parts in the death investigation sequence the Forensic Pathologist takes over. The Forensic Pathologist is a medical doctor who spends an additional 5 years specializing.
They are expertly trained to explore every possible cause of death.

It is a Forensic Pathologist who will sign off on cause of death. This is done through an autopsy. Every organ is dissected and examined for pathology, injury, poison, etc. Blood is drawn for toxicology. A decedent's pre-death health condition is ascertained to determine if it influenced the death of the individual.

A Forensic Pathologist will spend hours performing an autopsy. They will spend many more hours reviewing their findings. They have to review the bloodwork and toxicology. They have to evaluate any bodily trauma that may have been experienced. They will check and recheck their work to be certain they haven't missed any detail, no matter how small.

The Forensic Pathologist will review their findings with those of Law Enforcement first on the scene and that of the Forensic Investigator. The Forensic Pathologist will make sure there are no inconsistencies in the information as a cause of death conclusion is reached. As the Forensic Pathologist is so highly trained and his/her decision of cause of death is so important, the work involved and attention to detail they must provide is astounding. One erroneous conclusion as to cause of death can result in a murderer walking free, insurance fraud, lack of justice for the decedent and the decedent's family and need to exhume a body for re-evaluation. The pressure is intense, and the Forensic Pathologist faces this tough challenge perhaps thousands of times throughout their career. They are in charge of the Forensic case once it reaches the morgue. Their work is very strenuous, and their advanced training and credentialing brings them up to task. The Forensic Investigators, Forensic technicians, and Forensic Dentists play a subordinate role in the team that works death investigation at the morgue.

The Forensic Pathologist oversees the team. He/she determines what course of action is to be taken to determine cause of death. He/she determines if the cause of death was homicide, suicide, accidental, natural, unknown, or suspicious. The Forensic Pathologist can write cause of death and site the findings from autopsy, police reports, and Forensic Investigators. If the identity of a decedent is unknown there are several avenues a Forensic Pathologist can call upon. Fingerprints are very useful if the decedent has antemortem prints on file. Military personnel, Law Enforcement officers, and felons have prints on file as do many others. If there are no antemortem fingerprints on record a Forensic dentist can be called in. If the decedent has been to a dentist and had antemortem radiographs taken there is great likelihood postmortem dental examination with radiographs can be performed and a comparison study can be done. This can lead to identification. If this information is not available then DNA samples can be collected from the decedent and from a reliable antemortem source, such as the decedent's hairbrush. These can be compared for an identification. Prosthetic joints, tattoos, injuries, surgeries, age determinations, and birth defects can also aid in identification of a decedent. Some of these methods may not result in enough proof for an examiner to feel comfortable confirming an identification.

The Forensic Pathologist will decide when a Forensic Dentist's expertise is required. This request is common when there are no antemortem fingerprints on file. This is also the case when the condition of the decedent is damaged to the point that fingerprints cannot be acquired. This is commonly observed in fire victims or late term decomposition. The Forensic Pathologist forwards the information to the Forensic Investigator that the services of a Forensic Dentist are warranted. The Forensic Investigator connects with the Forensic Dentist and arranges for a postmortem dental examination with radiographs.

Without board certified Forensic Pathologists (Medical Examiners) death investigation would lose credibility and accuracy. There is a national shortage of these professionals.

I have had several interactions with Forensic Pathologists and Medical Examiners. They are highly intelligent, detail oriented people that are focused on providing a much-needed service to the community. They need a responsive sharp crew to work with.

There is a lot at stake with each death investigation, so they have to remain focused and have to record every detail.

Notes Chapter 2

Chapter 3

Chapter III.

Forensic dentist notification, materials, and supplies to bring, instruments used for examination, organization of workspace.

When it has been determined by the medical examiner that a decedent is required to have a scientific identification, the order is put out to contact the affiliated forensic dentist. This call can come at any time depending on the morgue with which the forensic dentist is affiliated. The busier and larger the morgue the more forensic dentists are available for contact. Forensic dentists can be called on an alternating schedule. In most identification cases it is sufficient to perform the examination after the dentist's regular workday. Occasionally there is a high priority need for the examination and identification to be completed as soon as possible so the dentist may need to reschedule his patients.

Once notified, the forensic dentist needs to make sure he/she has the necessary supplies and tools to complete the postmortem dental examination. I personally chose to buy a Black and Decker toolbox. It is sturdy, roomy, cleanable, and manageable. The kit contains the following:

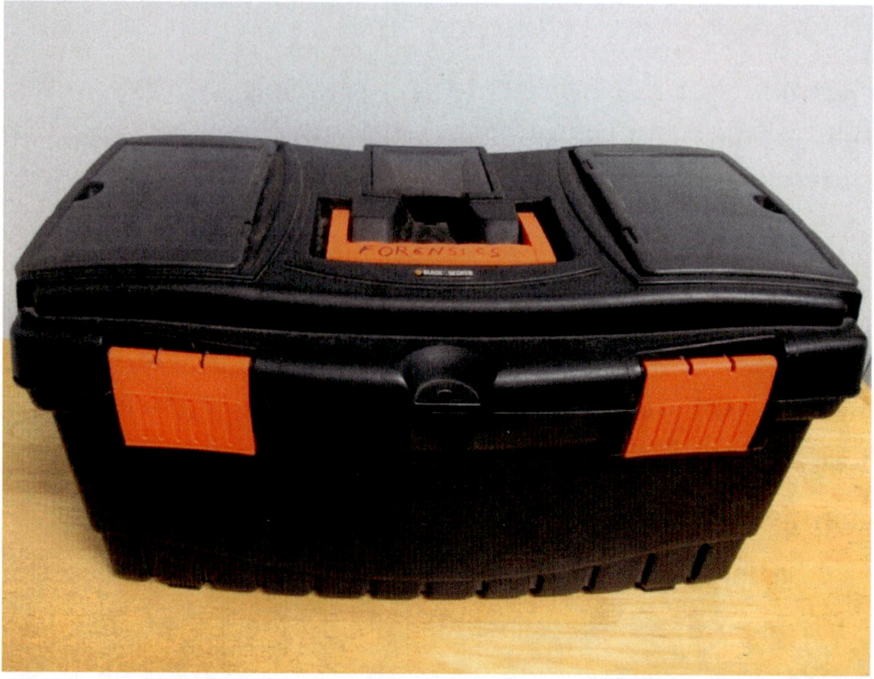

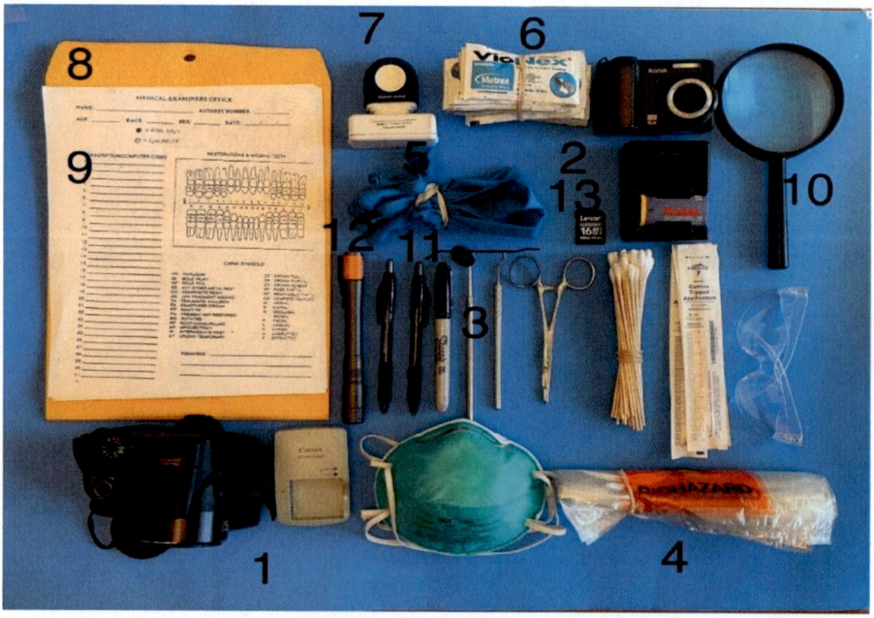

(Photographs of Black and Decker toolbox and contents)

1. Digital camera and charger
2. Spare digital camera and charger
3. Mirror and explorer
4. Evidence bags
5. Spare pairs of gloves
6. Alcohol wipes
7. Name stamp with line to sign name
8. Empty, large envelopes for paperwork for each case
9. Forensic dental examination sheet
10. Magnifying glass
11. Pens and markers
12. Flashlight
13. Spare SD cards for camera

Several of the above items are readily available at the morgue. I find it nice to carry extra supplies in case a supply issue arises. This ensures I would not be left in a position where my examination is compromised. As we will soon review, there are several additional supplies and tools that will be needed to complete a postmortem forensic dental examination. Together, this forensic kit represents a set up that has suited me well for over eighteen years. Additions or deletions of supplies can be expected form one forensic dentist to another. Updates or changes of supplies can also be expected.

The usual notification of a forensic dentist to come to the morgue to perform a postmortem forensic dental exam comes from a forensic investigator. They are hardworking people exposed to very traumatic, horrific events. They see people in the worst possible conditions and witness what people are capable of doing to each other. The (non-forensic) typical person may experience this type of traumatic exposure once in a lifetime and be traumatized for life over it. Investigators, (think about this) see these events *thousands* of times over the course of their careers. I like to keep this in mind as they call me. No matter how hectic my day, if I am tired, if I have to change my plans day or night, or if I have personal things to tend to, I make every effort to be as friendly, accommodating, helpful, humble, and polite as possible. My choice of behavior may be the only, nice interaction this investigator will experience all day. It is important to treat them with respect. You can make allies and friends with a decent attitude. Courtesy goes a long way.

If you have a staff member in your regular dental practice who has expressed an interest in forensics, consider yourself fortunate. Through your access to forensics you can share your knowledge with them as they in turn help you with packing the equipment, organization, the examination, write up, x-ray development, and any other follow through that may be necessary in your case. I have been fortunate to have dental assistants from my general practice that share a strong interest in forensic dentistry. They carefully prepare the toolbox and equipment for a case and accompany me to the morgue. Having someone hit the exposure button on the x ray machine, chart the information on the teeth, and document the case as I dictate greatly reduces the complexities of the exam and eases the burden of juggling all the aspects involved. The decedents are often in a condition where a second set of hands is more than useful to gather the information needed to make a dental identification. My assistants also print and label the digital photographs taken during a dental identification case. I record the body identification tag and take one to several photographs of the decedent. Photographs can aid in recollection of the case years later. Photographs can also aid in the understanding of why radiographs may look atypical. An example is a shotgun suicide when the shot is fired in the mouth and fractures to the mandible and maxilla result.

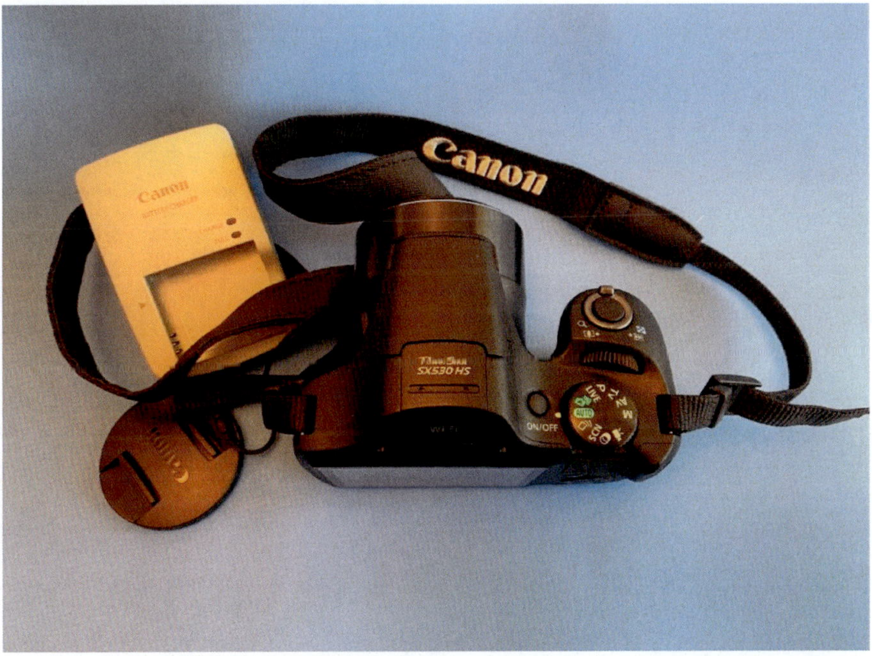

(Photograph of current camera)

As a forensic dentist I have found the vast majority of identification is accomplished via the dental radiographs; antemortem radiographs compared to the postmortem radiographs. Digital photographs are a useful adjunct to formulate your final assessment of the identification.

Originally, I used the old system of duplicate radiographs. They were "taken," exposed, and the protective casings were opened in a darkroom and the radiographs were fed through a chemical processor. They were dried then mounted in a "radiograph photo album" of sorts. They were read and comparison studies were made against available antemortem radiographs.

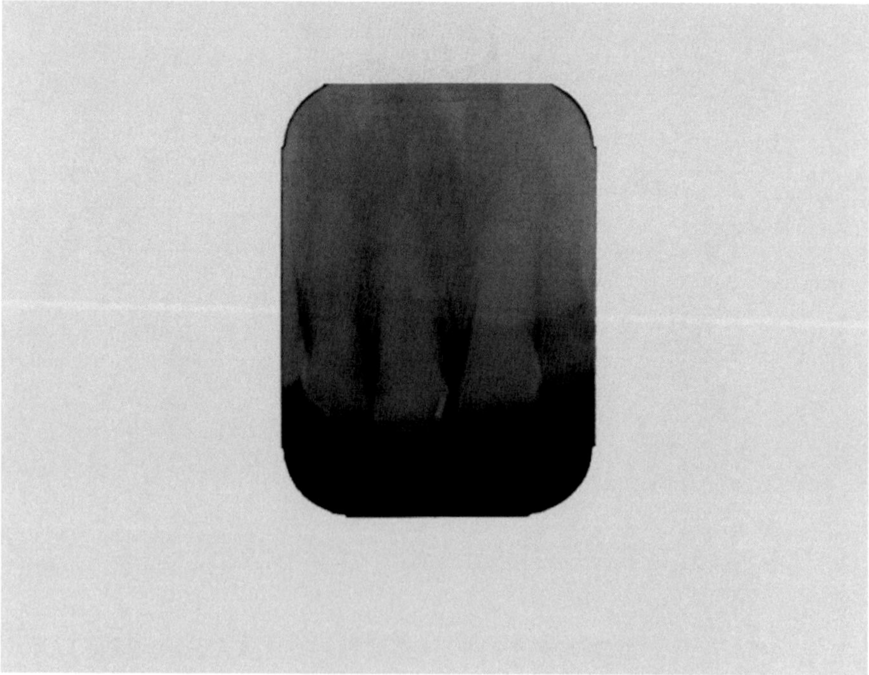

(1)

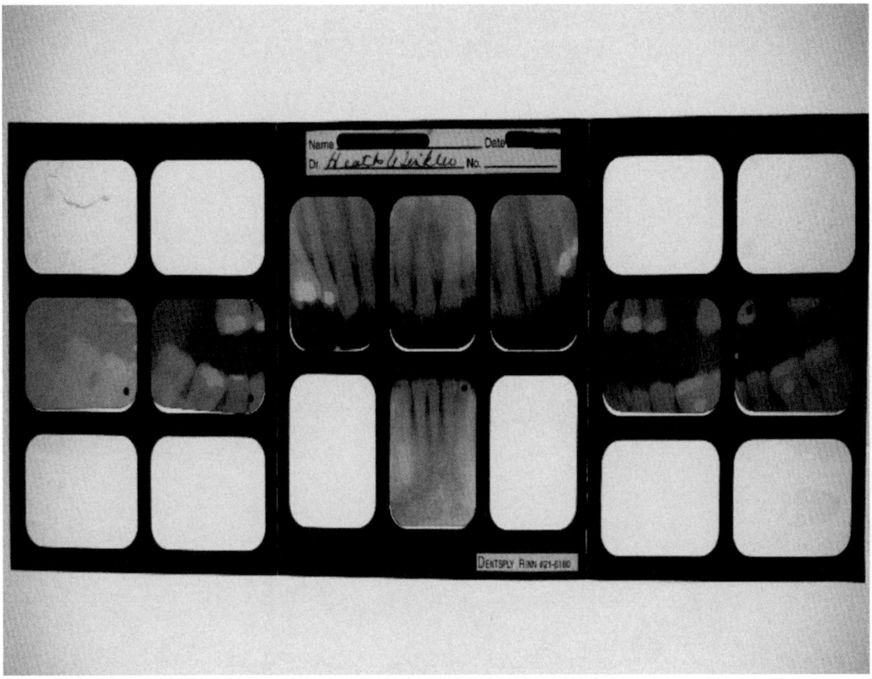

(2)

1. Photograph of chemically processed radiographs
2. Mounted chemically processed radiographs

Around 2015 I was able to upgrade to phosphor plates. A darkroom wasn't needed. However, they were still very light sensitive so minimal exposure to light was important. These were "exposed," and the protective sheath was removed. The exposed phosphor plates are mounted into a processing unit and uploaded into a computer program. They can then be sorted, arranged appropriately, and printed on photopaper for examination.

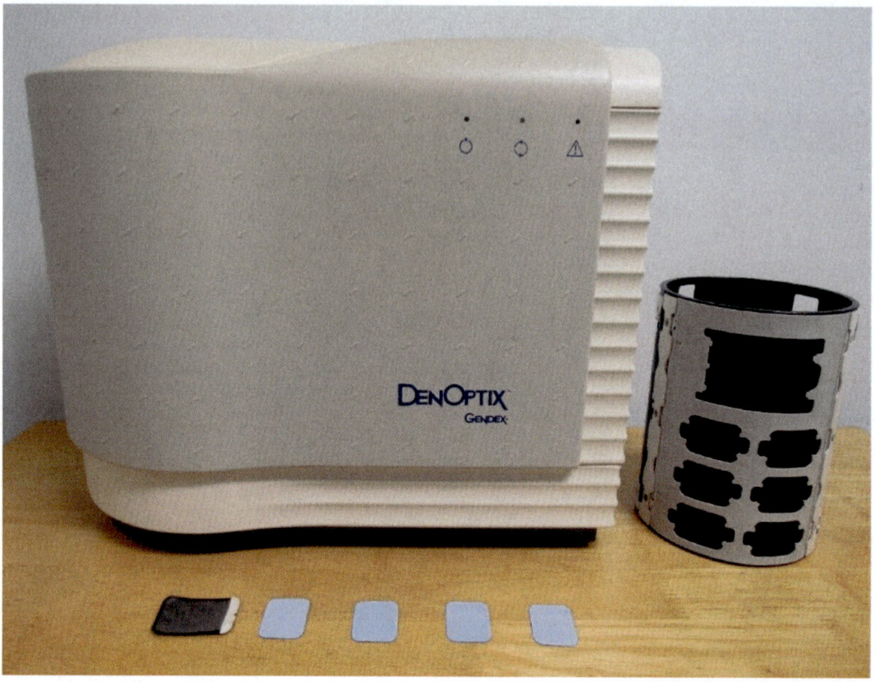

(Photograph of Phosphor Plate Radiograph System)

Both of these radiographic systems served me well over the years. They both provided accurate detail which I could reliably use to draw conclusions on postmortem dental identification cases. The biggest drawback with both systems was not having developed radiographs in hand that day. There was always the worry that the exposure didn't work correctly, or the processor may ruin the radiographs. It was impractical to bring the developers to the morgue, so you had to wait to process and review the radiographs at your private office. That meant two round trips to the morgue for every case. A worse case possibility was that your radiographs didn't turn out well and the morgue released the decedent's body after you performed your examination. Family and funeral homes are waiting to start their roles in the process, and it would be awkward at the very least, to recall a released decedent so you could take new radiographs.

This brings me to the system I utilize now. It is a fully digital system. It can be integrated with the internet, but I chose to keep it offline, and this makes it an independent system which cannot be compromised by hackers. After I am done printing the radiographs, I simply write the case number on the radiographs with a pen; no identification to hack into; no internet to compromise. (A side note: when I was a military officer, my information was hacked into at the Department of Defense level. Enemies of the U.S. were targeting all military officers and their families. I do not trust the internet's users and I do as much of my private practice, forensics and private life offline as possible).

I wanted that ability to print radiographs right at the morgue. I bought the smallest printer/copier I could find and mounted the laptop to it. I also purchased a rugged duffle bag that is waterproof for easy cleanup. Now I can pack everything up at my general office, load my vehicle, and head to the morgue knowing I can print my radiographs.

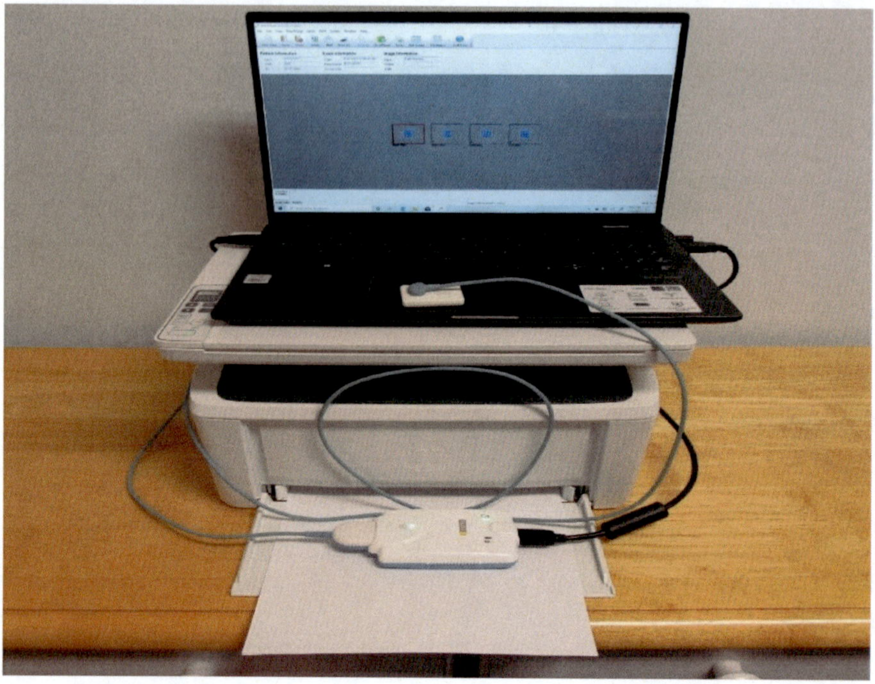

(Photograph of Digital X-ray System)

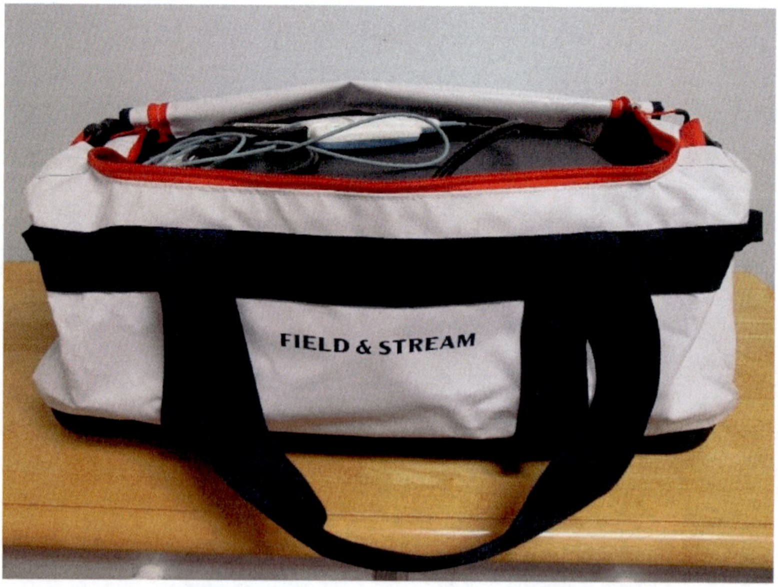

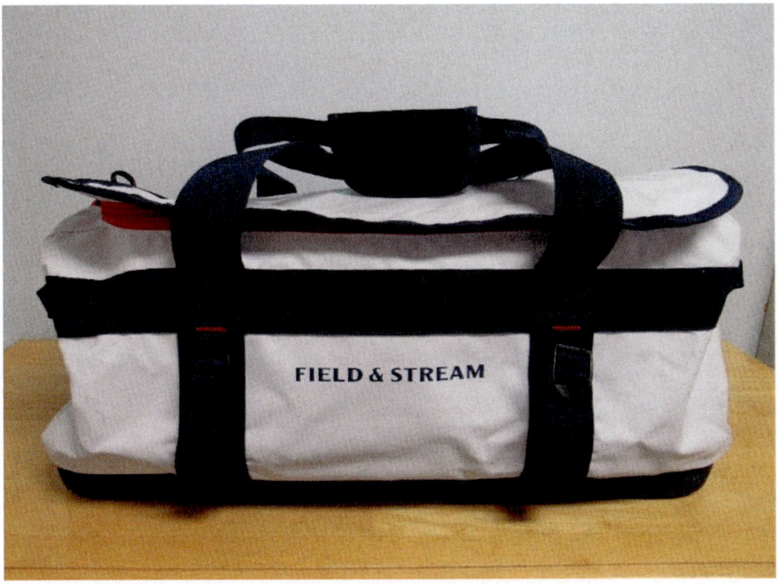

(Photographs of Digital X-ray System, Printer & Carrying Bag)

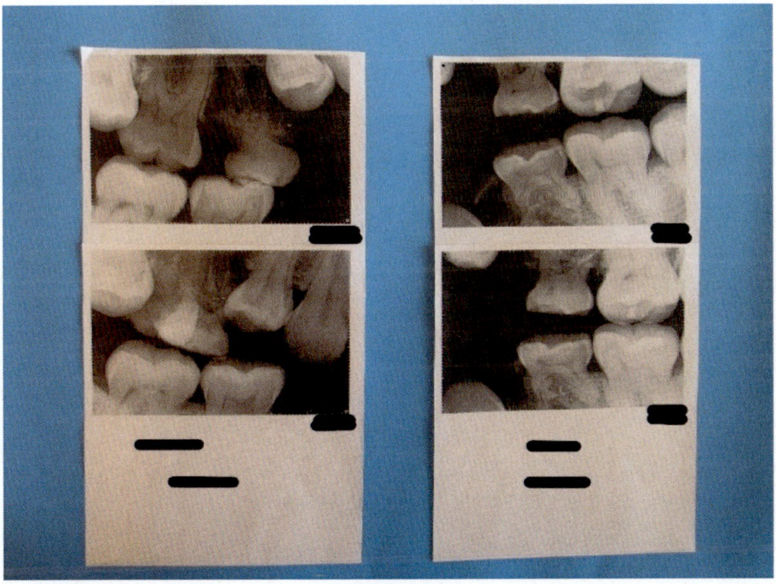

(Photograph of Postmortem Radiographs)

With the vehicle packed, the trip is made to the morgue. Security at the morgue requires you to be checked in by security personnel, to get into the parking lot and then the lobby. The morgue deals with the remains of loved ones which is very emotional. The emotional state of loved ones can escalate and create potential harmful/dangerous situations. This is not a place to leave accessible to adventuresome or opportunistic individuals. Having security measures are a must.

Once through security, the forensic dentist waits for a forensic investigator escort to be let into the autopsy or special autopsy room.

Before entering the autopsy or special autopsy room, there is a room for your items you do not want exposed to be safely stored until you have completed the exam. Usually, the later at night you go the quieter the morgue. I personally prefer later at night to avoid peak city traffic and to have a less chaotic and congested morgue to work in. This situation can vary based on circumstances but generally holds true.

In the hallway outside the autopsy rooms is a cart which contains various safety barriers for you to utilize while performing the postmortem forensic dental examination. These barriers can all be used, or you can pick your personal comfort level based on the condition of the decedent.

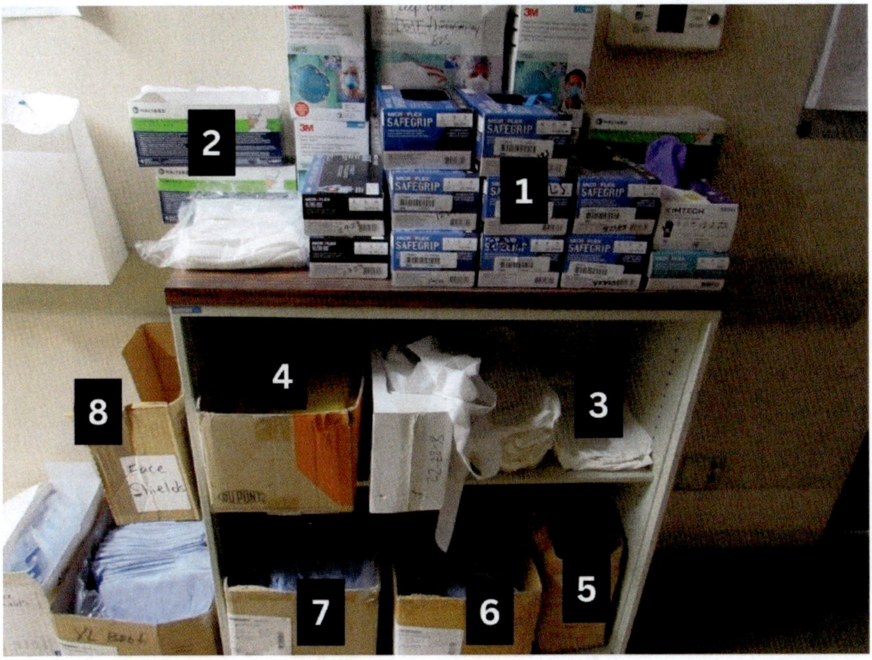

(Photograph of Forensic Barriers Cart in Hallway)

1. Gloves, heavy duty
2. Mask
3. Sleeve guards
4. Apron
5. Gown
6. Booties
7. Hairnet
8. Face shield

Once you have donned the proper attire you can enter the autopsy room. There you will find a small toolbox containing applicable dental tools.

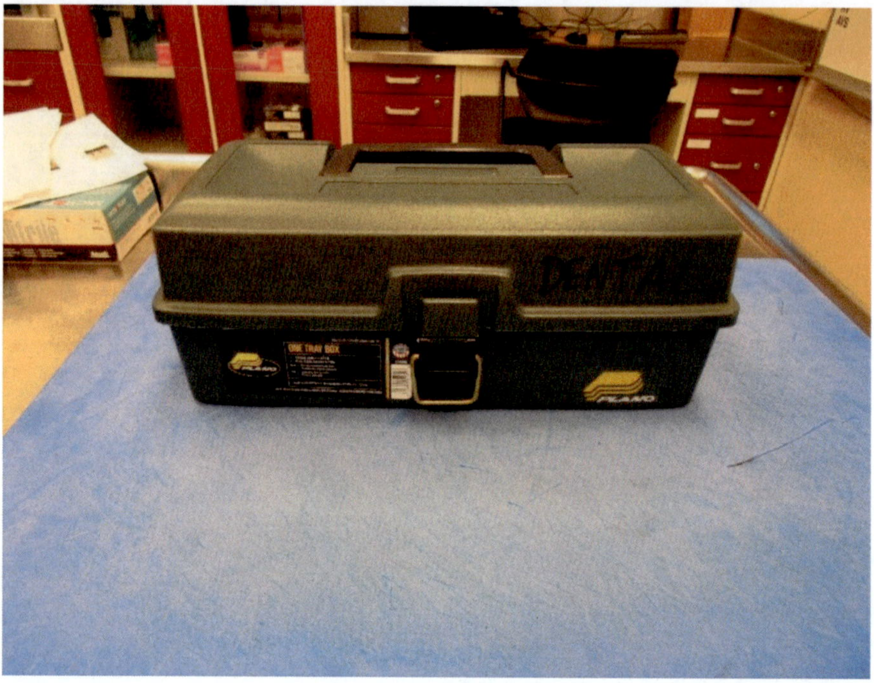

(Photograph of Dental Toolbox Supplied by the Morgue)

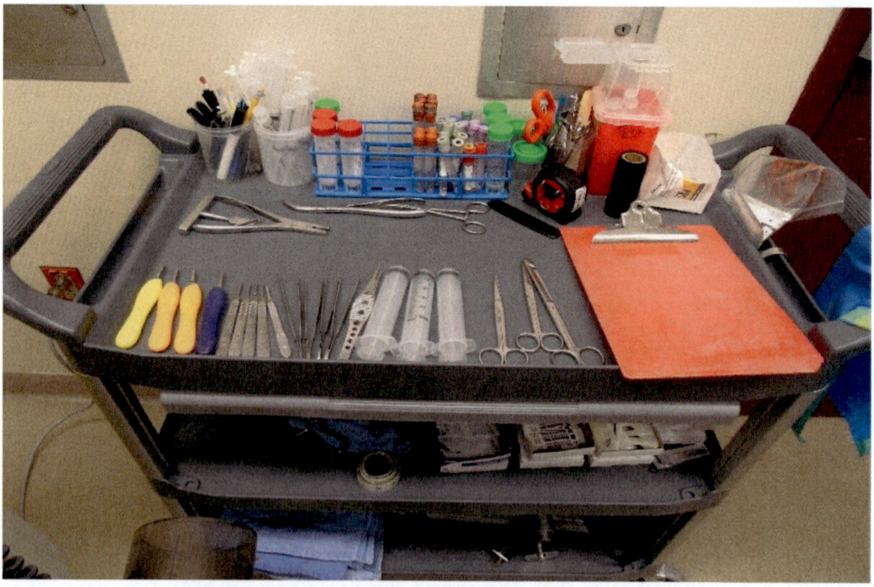

(Photograph of Autopsy Cart)

There is also an autopsy cart that has several useful items for forensic dental examinations.

Having access to your own forensic toolbox, the supplied toolbox, and items from the autopsy cart you can set up for your forensic dental examination. I typically set up the digital radiography equipment first. I will take radiographs after I look at the decedent's oral cavity to see which radiographic exposures will be the most useful in determining their identity.

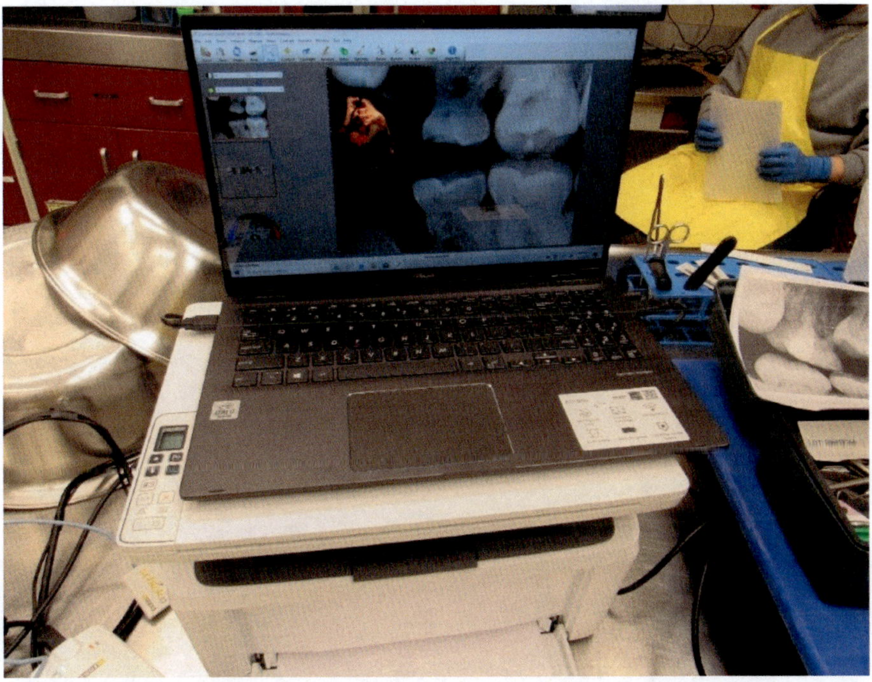

(Photograph of digital radiography equipment set up and ready for use at the morgue)

You will need to take as many radiographs as is necessary to draw identification conclusions. If you know ahead of time the antemortem dental radiograph of the decedent available is a PA of #11 (upper left canine) a full mouth series of postmortem radiographs will not be of use except for radiographs showing #11. The number of postmortem dental radiographs taken can vary based on the condition of the decedent. This will be discussed case by case in future chapters. Antemortem charting can also be compared to both postmortem radiographs and postmortem charting for consistencies.

Once the dental radiographs are in place, you should have the forensic dental toolbox, autopsy cart, and your own forensic dental toolbox within easy reach of your working area. You may also have access to a portable x-ray unit, as shown below:

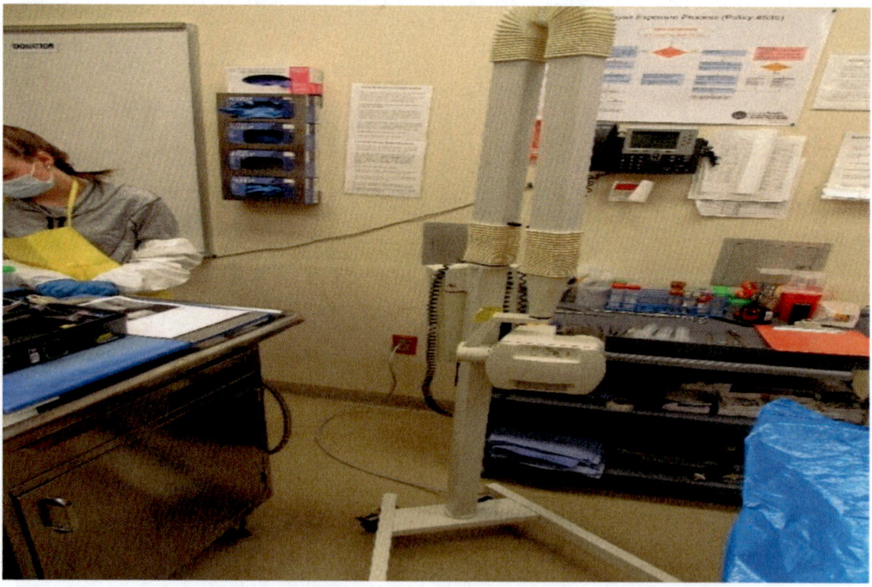

At this point you are ready for the decedent. Typical cases where the body is intact will have the bodies in the main autopsy room cooler. Cases of mutilation, severe burns, explosions, decomp, etc. will be in the special autopsy room cooler. Frequently the latter will be the cases for the forensic dentist and his/her examinations will take place in the special autopsy room.

You should make every effort to help the forensic investigator or technician retrieve the decedent. Decedents are on a stainless steel gurney in a body bag. These gurneys are cumbersome to steer, and they need to go through sets of doors. It makes the investigator's job a little easier if you pitch in and help with the gurney or at least open the doors.

Once the decedent is at your work area you should take a photograph of the ID tag on the body bag. Next, the body bag can be opened and, if applicable, the headrest can be removed from under the decedent's head. Photographs can be taken before, during, or after the postmortem forensic dental examination depending on what needs to be documented and if the sequence is important. For example, if you are recording the sequence of events for a facial dissection you have to take before, during, and after photographs since you are altering the decedent irreversibly.

Hopefully you will have a technician, forensic investigator, or your assistant to help you chart, take photographs, and press the button for radiographic exposures. This saves a tremendous amount of running back and forth and contaminating charts, cameras, and various other forensic tools. If you work alone you would have to re-glove every time you go from direct contact with the decedent to your camera, chart, or instrument box to prevent contamination from the decedent to your equipment and tools.

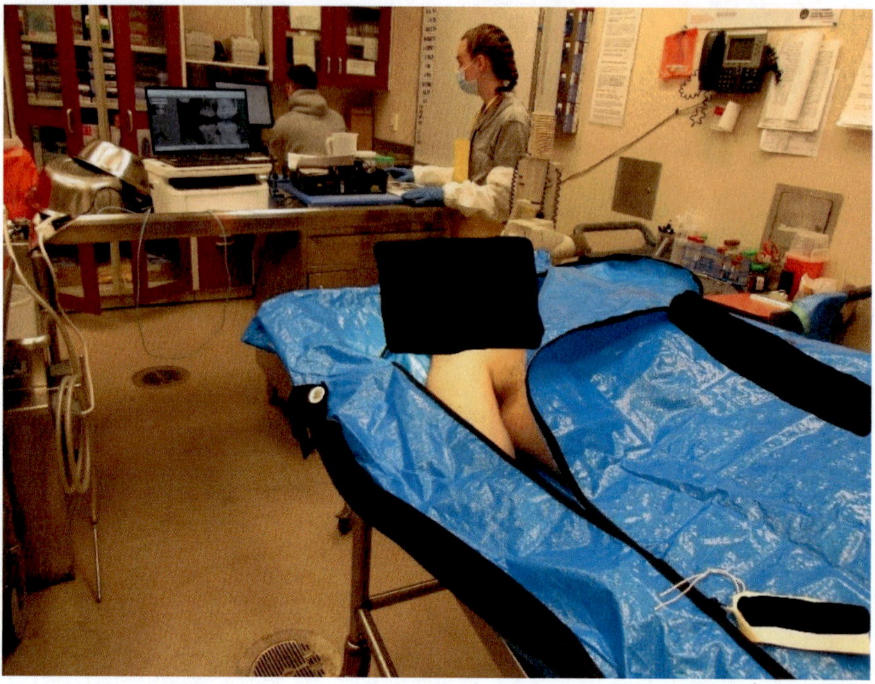

An example of a postmortem forensic dental examination with an investigator, assistant, and the decedent. The toolbox, radiographic equipment and supplemental tools are also available for use.

I have recently upgraded my radiographic equipment to a Nomad 2 pro system. It is much easier to expose radiographic images with it and far less cumbersome. I no longer need to wheel the portable x-ray unit in and put it away after use.

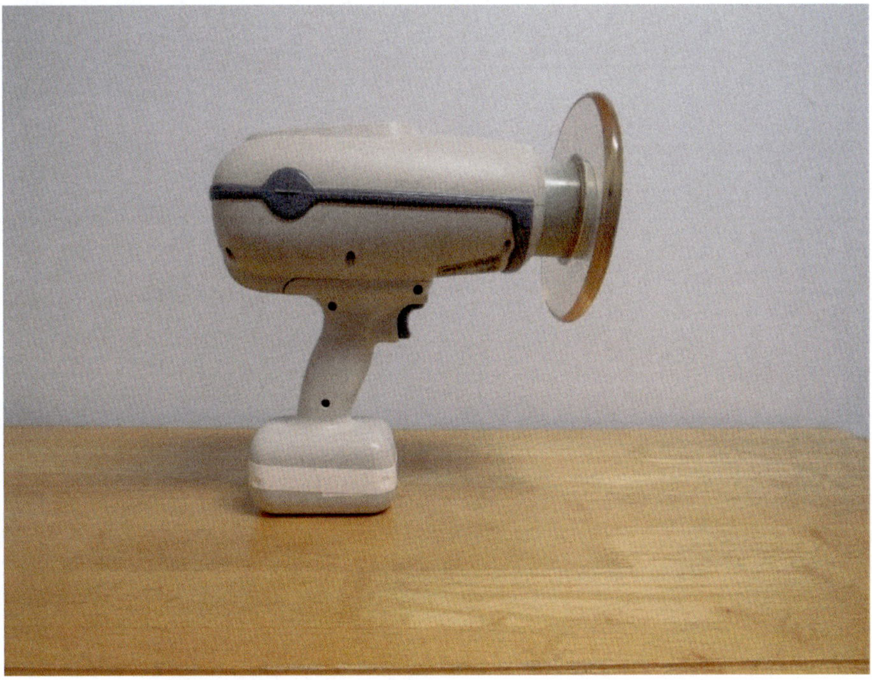

(Photograph of the Nomad 2 pro)

Notes Chapter Three

Chapter 4

Chapter IV.

Intended goals of postmortem forensic dental examination, radiographs, photographs, charting anomalies, unique feature.

The photographs of the decedent are sometimes taken throughout the examination. Here the forensic dentist is given the challenges of dealing with a decedent that can be very difficult and challenging to work with. Burn victims may require facial dissection to access the oral cavity. Victims of mass trauma may require you to reconstruct to the best of your ability some type of resemblance to a maxilla and mandible. You may have to clean the oral cavity of blood, maggots, decomposing flesh, or insects. Whatever the condition of the decent your goal as a forensic dentist is to be as attentive as possible to every detail. Next, record those details and use that information to make comparisons to corresponding antemortem records. It is not good practice to review antemortem records prior to conducting your postmortem dental examination as this examination could bias your opinion. It can persuade you to perhaps draw a certain conclusion you may not otherwise come to. Do not put the cart before the horse. Look at the antemortem dental records and do your comparison studies after you have completed your postmortem dental examination with charting, radiographs, and photographs. It is ok to make updated entries on your charting as long as you label it as such and date the information accordingly. One exception I have made over the years is to look at the antemortem dental radiographs that are available. I do not review the teeth. I merely see what radiographs I need to take for comparison. For example, if one set of four bitewings is available for antemortem records I would take four postmortem bitewings. I usually will not bother with a full mouth series of postmortem radiographs because I would have nothing to compare them to. One may argue an FMX would be more prudent. You could take one. Keep in mind you also want to be efficient. Common sense may lead you to take one or two extra PAs of a tooth exhibiting an easily identifiable restoration or anatomical anomaly. Do what is efficient and necessary to properly conduct your examination.

Charting of the teeth in the United States starts with the upper back right most tooth(wisdom) as tooth #1 and goes to the upper left wisdom tooth as #16. You then drop to the lower left wisdom tooth and call it #17. You move along to the bottom right wisdom tooth and call it #32. This is for adult dentiton. Each tooth keeps its number even if there are other teeth missing. Primary teeth are 20 in number. However, they are labeled A though T. They also start with the upper right (As A) and end up at lower right with tooth letter T.

This is important to understand. Other countries use different charting systems which will not align with the U.S. system. Instead of #1 through #32, you will experience such systems as using ┘,L,┐,Γ with numbers. The symbols signify quadrants (upper right, upper left, lower right, and lower left respectively). The numbers will be 1-8 for each tooth per quadrant. An example is the upper right 3rd tooth from the front. The U.S. system would call the tooth #6. It is not important to memorize different charting systems. It is important to recognize where the antemortem records came from and to research how that system works.

Radiographs in the U.S. are viewed as if you are looking at the person face to face. Some countries view radiographs as if you are sitting in the mouth looking out. This is important as the radiographs will be backwards. Beware of these possibilities and act accordingly. Restorations, tooth rotations, decay, tilts, missing teeth, diastemas, and types of restorative materials are recorded as carefully as possible. Teeth often need to be cleaned and recleaned as you perform your examination due to oozing fluids, blood, maggot migration, shot or any other of a variety of visual obstructions. Information is best verbalized to an assistant who will chart for you. They will record your findings for you. Working alone requires you to glove and unglove several times during an exam so as not to contaminate the charts and make a mess. Your dental examination will be transferred onto a chart for later comparison.

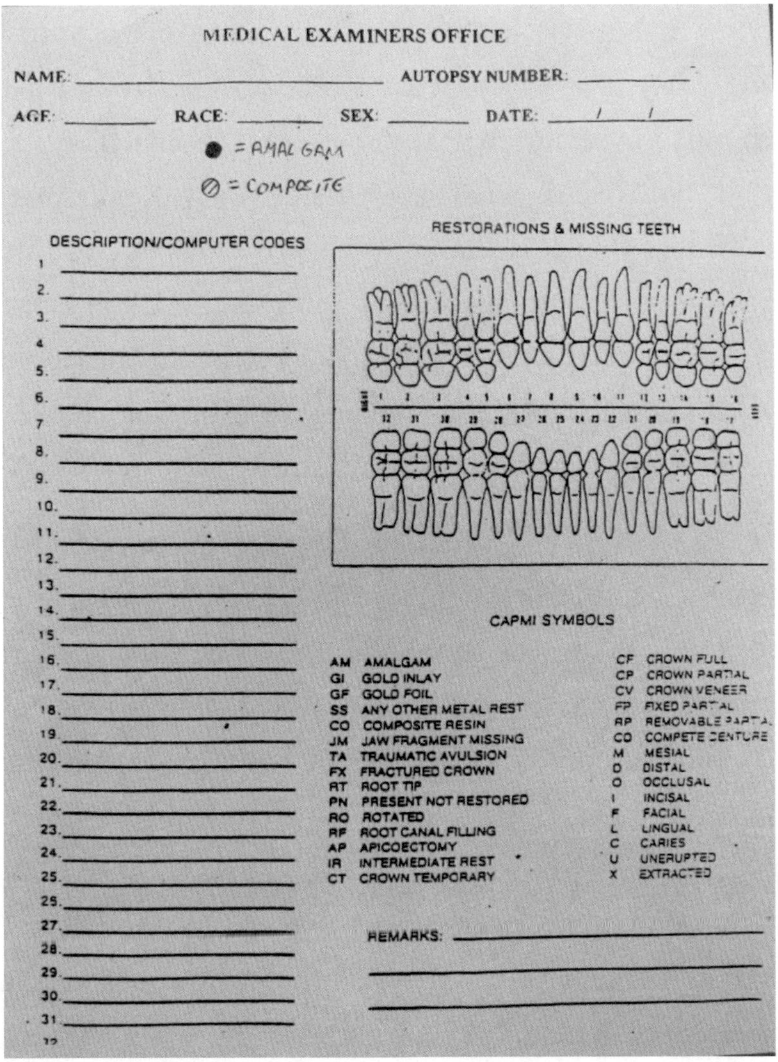

MEDICAL EXAMINERS OFFICE

NAME: ____________ AUTOPSY NUMBER: ____________

AGE: ________ RACE: ________ SEX: ________ DATE: ___/___/___

● = AMALGAM

⊘ = COMPOSITE

DESCRIPTION/COMPUTER CODES

1. ____
2. ____
3. ____
4. ____
5. ____
6. ____
7. ____
8. ____
9. ____
10. ____
11. ____
12. ____
13. ____
14. ____
15. ____
16. ____
17. ____
18. ____
19. ____
20. ____
21. ____
22. ____
23. ____
24. ____
25. ____
25. ____
27. ____
28. ____
29. ____
30. ____
31. ____

RESTORATIONS & MISSING TEETH

CAPMI SYMBOLS

AM	AMALGAM	CF	CROWN FULL
GI	GOLD INLAY	CP	CROWN PARTIAL
GF	GOLD FOIL	CV	CROWN VENEER
SS	ANY OTHER METAL REST	FP	FIXED PARTIAL
CO	COMPOSITE RESIN	RP	REMOVABLE PARTIAL
JM	JAW FRAGMENT MISSING	CD	COMPETE DENTURE
TA	TRAUMATIC AVULSION	M	MESIAL
FX	FRACTURED CROWN	D	DISTAL
RT	ROOT TIP	O	OCCLUSAL
PN	PRESENT NOT RESTORED	I	INCISAL
RO	ROTATED	F	FACIAL
RF	ROOT CANAL FILLING	L	LINGUAL
AP	APICOECTOMY	C	CARIES
IR	INTERMEDIATE REST	U	UNERUPTED
CT	CROWN TEMPORARY	X	EXTRACTED

REMARKS: ____________

(Photograph of charting with additional key to improve conveyance of information)

If you wish to make additional notes or record more information, you can do so on your charting. I like to add the key you can see in the photograph. It allows me to easily relay the type of restorative material used on the decedent and recorded in the postmortem dental exam. I also write a note stating, "x-rays to be reviewed" and follow that up with signed and dated notes on the postmortem charting after the postmortem radiographs are reviewed. If radiographs are reviewed at the same time as charting the "to be reviewed" notes on the chart are not necessary. Remember this is a postmortem dental examination chart so do not add notes or change information on it from antemortem dental radiographs or from antemortem dental progress notes. The timeline would be off in the postmortem dental charting update. The chart is for postmortem information and details only.

When you are finished with charting your postmortem findings you sign the postmortem dental chart and make sure all dates are correct. I have a forensic stamp that I use since my signature may be difficult to read. My assistant will also sign the postmortem dental examination. Investigators and technicians do not care to sign off on the charting that they assisted. I make a copy of the postmortem charts for my records and stamp that it is indeed a copy. This stamped copy is kept in the forensic dentist's case file and the original is given to the attending forensic investigator or forensic technician.

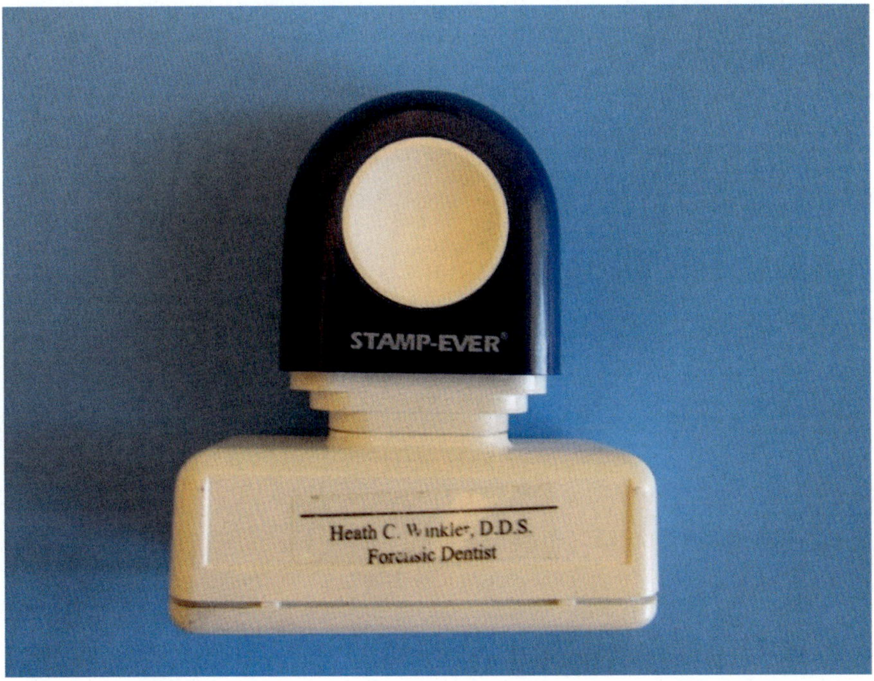

(Forensic Dentist stamp to be used with postmortem charting and on the forensic identification write up.)

You should feel like you have given it your best effort to compile enough information in the postmortem dental examination to make good solid correlations with the antemortem records. The more detailed information you have observed and recorded the better.

Good radiographs are paramount to a solid comparison study. Taking radiographs can be challenging depending on the condition of the decedent. Generally, I tend to fill the mouth with paper towels. The tongue is removed during most autopsies. Any void remaining in the oral cavity filled up by paper towels is now solid enough to keep radiographs steady. Fill the empty space and stabilize the radiographs in the mouth. I like to place radiographs in the mouth with hemostats, get them positioned correctly, and remove the hemostats prior to exposing the radiograph.

Throughout the postmortem dental examination, it is important to pay attention to details. Anything that stands out during the examination as out of line, unusual, or unique should be documented and charted. Take your time with the postmortem dental examination. You will often be challenged with contamination in the oral cavity. Keep your work area as clean as possible by wiping the oral cavity with gauze and paper towels. Pressing into the teeth with an explorer, it can sometimes expose what you think is decay or a restoration as a piece of debris or vice versa. As with any human being, you will be prone to make mistakes every now and then. It is a fact of life that can be hard to live with. If you are in error, it is best to take your lumps immediately, own your error, and remedy it as best as you can. At the very least you have addressed the situation honestly and honorably. It is not easy to do but in the long run it is the best way to conduct yourself and you can maintain your integrity. You will know your own words will hold value. Mistakes made in record taking, involve an initialed, single line through the error. The correct information added should be dated and initiated by the individual doing the correction.

I make corrections to my postmortem forensic charting when warranted. As mentioned earlier, I will complete the examination and write a note on the chart stating, "x-rays to be reviewed." In the next day or so I review the radiographs and often find several new chartable bits of information. For example, unerupted wisdom teeth are marked with an "X" in the charting. There is no ability to see unerupted teeth without radiographs, so I simply make a note stating "#1, #16, #17, #32 were observed on radiographs." I sign and date the change and write "unerupted" above the wisdom teeth on the visual chart. There may be occasions where a well-placed composite is missed on an exam but shows up on radiographs. I change PN (present, not restored) to (i.e.) #29-O comp. It would look like the following:

#27 PN____

#28 PN____

HW

#29 ~~PN~~ O-Comp

#30 PN____

#31 PN____

As was mentioned earlier, I now use digital radiography. I can view the postmortem radiographs as I complete the postmortem dental charting. I can make corrections and updates to the records much sooner.

At this point you are ready to see the antemortem dental records of the tentative decedent and start your comparison studies. If there are no antemortem dental records available at this point, you are finished for the evening. You make a case file for yourself and hold onto the file until further notice. This may be in a day or two or it could be the end of this case if there are no antemortem dental records available. This does happen as older records are destroyed, or the decedent never visited a dentist, or there is no idea who the decedent is, and the decedent's dentist is unknown for contact.

Notes Chapter Four

Chapter 5

Chapter V.

Conclusions, forensic write up, guidelines for conveying your examination.

At this point of the examination, you will be given the entire postmortem forensic file on the decedent which includes the antemortem dental information. You also have all of your information; charting, notes, and radiographs acquired during your postmortem dental examination.

I like to use the library at the morgue to lay out all the paperwork on a large table. It is nice to be able to have information spread out so you can see everything at once instead of constantly shuffling through papers and radiographs. Available workspace obviously depends on where you are working. Try to set yourself up where it is quiet and comfortable.

I first review the written antemortem dental charting. There can be useful information contained in the antemortem charting that you may otherwise miss. An example could be if it is in the written notes that #6 is rotated 90 degrees. This helps because there are no antemortem radiographs of #6, just bitewings. Consequently, I only took bitewings, but I recorded the rotation of #6 in the postmortem dental examination. The findings are consistent. This can be recorded in the postmortem dental examination write up to help strengthen my conclusion.

I next take the postmortem radiographs and set them on the table adjacent to the antemortem radiographs. This is when I go through tooth by tooth. I check that corresponding teeth are present in both sets of radiographs. If a tooth is only there on one set of radiographs, it has to be present on the antemortem films. The assumption is the tooth was lost between the antemortem radiographs and the postmortem radiographs. We cannot grow teeth postmortem so, if it is the other way around, you have reason for concern.

The opposite order of events goes for decay, amalgams, composites, root canals, and crowns. They can all be in postmortem radiographs but not in antemortem radiographs. The timeline of events makes sense. It has to. It helps to ask yourself the right questions: Could this be here before life ended but be missing after life ended? Could this situation be present in death but not be present in life? Confirming your postmortem dental information and your antemortem dental information fall into place sequentially is what you need to accomplish to have a sound argument in your comparison studies.

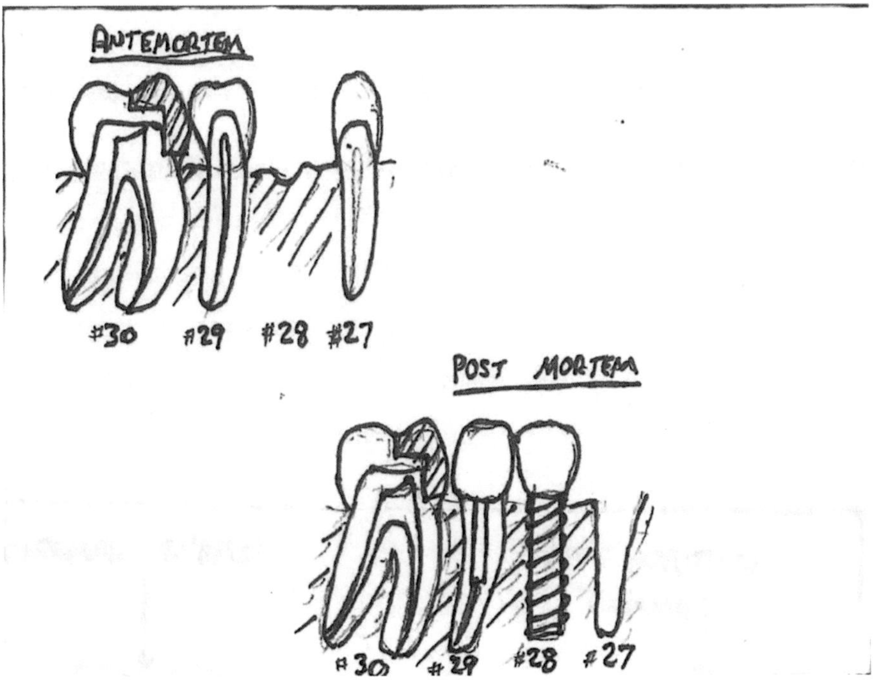

(Illustration of post mortem & antemortem radiographs)

A) #30 could have an antemortem MO composite that is present in the postmortem radiographs

B) #29 could be a virgin tooth structure in antemortem radiographs and could have subsequently had a RCT, post, and crown.

C) #28 cannot be missing in an antemortem radiograph and be present in a postmortem radiograph. It could present as an implant or a pontic on a fixed bridge in a postmortem radiograph

D) #27 can be present in an antemortem radiograph and absent in a postmortem radiograph.

A, B, C, D, are all reasonable courses of events from antemortem to postmortem. For #28, the decedent had an implant placed.

One must ask the question: is this possible without a time machine? This sounds a bit childish but can be effective. Each tooth that presents differently in the antemortem radiographs and postmortem radiographs is held accountable to a timeline. A tooth cannot appear after you are dead. Restorations can be placed after a set of living radiographs and before death. A tooth can be removed that was in a living person's radiographs. It can consequently be missing in radiographs after the same person's death. Your goals are to find consistency and make sure everything makes sense in a timeline.

Large amalgam restorations and root canals are very helpful in identification. The more the better. Pay attention to the shape of the tooth, crown, the root, and the restoration. Decide if the variations in radiograph angulations can be accounted for when the shape is not exact upon antemortem radiograph and postmortem radiograph analysis and comparison.

If there are a few, or even no restorations in a decedent's dentition, the complexity of the comparison increases. This is where you need to start looking at bone levels and density, pulp horns, root morphology, attrition patterns, cuspal anatomy, and tilting or rotating of teeth. This is what you will need to complete comparison studies. Comparisons of many areas need to be noted in these cases to make a strong case.

The more the above listed categories match up, the less likely the decedent is someone other than who you are assuming it is.

Write up your postmortem dental examination findings as you see them. Do not try to make pieces of the puzzle fit together by pushing or stretching what is observed. Actual observed and recorded facts are what a forensic dentist is there to gather. If there is not enough evidence to come to a conclusion, then that needs to be stated. A forensic dentist needs to follow scientific protocol to the best of their ability.

When I write up a case, I state what I see. Nothing more. Nothing less. If it is a routine case and there are several good restorations and good, clear postmortem radiographs and antemortem radiographs I would review and document that the post and antemortem radiographs are consistent. I would also bring attention to areas of interest. For example, if there was a four surface amalgam on #30 with many unique features and shapes consistent on each set of radiographs I would write:

Special areas of interest include the MODB amalgam on #30." The more areas of consistency you mention the better your case presents.

In a case where there is not much to work with in a restorative sense, I actually take out a large magnifying glass and review the teeth, bone, and sinuses. Sinus shapes and their intimacy with root apices can aid in identification. Bone density, bone level, type of bone loss (acute or chronic), and location of the inferior alveolar nerve in relation to the root apices and location in the mandible can aid in diagnosis. Root orientation, morphology, canal shapes, pulp horn configurations, and wear patterns can be utilized. Whatever you can observe and document that helps draw a conclusion should be studied and noted in your postmortem forensic dental examination.

As I write up a case, I look at the evidence in front of me. Each consistency is multiplied by the others to draw a conclusion. It would be extremely difficult if not impossible to put an exact number (comparisons) on a likelihood.

You can come up with conservative numbers and you will see confidence increases with each added observation.

If you have 4 antemortem dental radiographs and 4 postmortem dental radiographs for comparison and you apply ultraconservative probabilities to the conditions seen in each set of radiographs you can see how a non-match quickly becomes extremely remote.

Odds of mod amalgam on #29 with same shape 1/50	Odds of #14 with angular bone loss 1/2	Odds of having an impacted #6 1/10	Odds of same canal morphology 2,3,4,5 1/60
Odds of same attrition patterns #32 1/10	Odds of MIL Chip #8 1/10	Odds of MIL Chip #9 1/10	

I have given an example of recording 7 consistencies between postmortem radiographs and antemortem radiographs. The ultra-conservative odds of these radiographs being from 2 different people are:

1/50 x 1/2x 1/10x 1/60x 1/10x 1/10x 1/10 = 1/60,000,000

Chances of a coincidental exact match of two different people becomes remote fairly quickly. That being said, there is still a chance here. That is why I write "consistent." Writing up a case with this many comparisons that match and remembering that I use very conservative odds, gives the consistent conclusion to forensic dental identification cases credibility.

We have reviewed a forensic dentist's interactions with his/her affiliated morgue. We have discussed the forensic investigator, the Medical Examiner, and several other key persons in the chain of forensic identification. We have reviewed equipment, forensic thought process and protocols. We discussed manners and teamwork. The next several chapters of the book will contain actual examples, with photographs, of cases I have completed. Cause of death will be reviewed as well as what considerations need to be addressed in post mortem examination based on decedent condition in order to collect the information that is needed in the postmortem Forensic Dental examination.

Notes Chapter Five

Chapter 6

Chapter VI.
Decomposition

There are decomposition cases where fingerprints are not available for recording and comparison. Fingerprints decompose over time resulting in distortion and deletion of information within the fingerprint. Identification becomes impossible. Also, a decedent may have never had their fingerprints recorded making a comparison impossible.

Teeth, on the other hand, are far more durable and resistant to degradation. The human body can be in any of several stages of decomposition and the teeth will be in fine shape for identification. In this chapter we will review several examples and stages of decomposition and the teeth will be in fine shape for identification. In this chapter we will review several examples and stages of decomposition and considerations for each case when performing a postmortem forensic dental examination. The goal is common; a thorough fact finding, detailed examination. You will find out how collecting this information will take different levels of effort based on the condition of the subject.

Decomposition in water after a drowning or someone dumping a body in water after death will expose you to the similarities and differences of land decomposition.

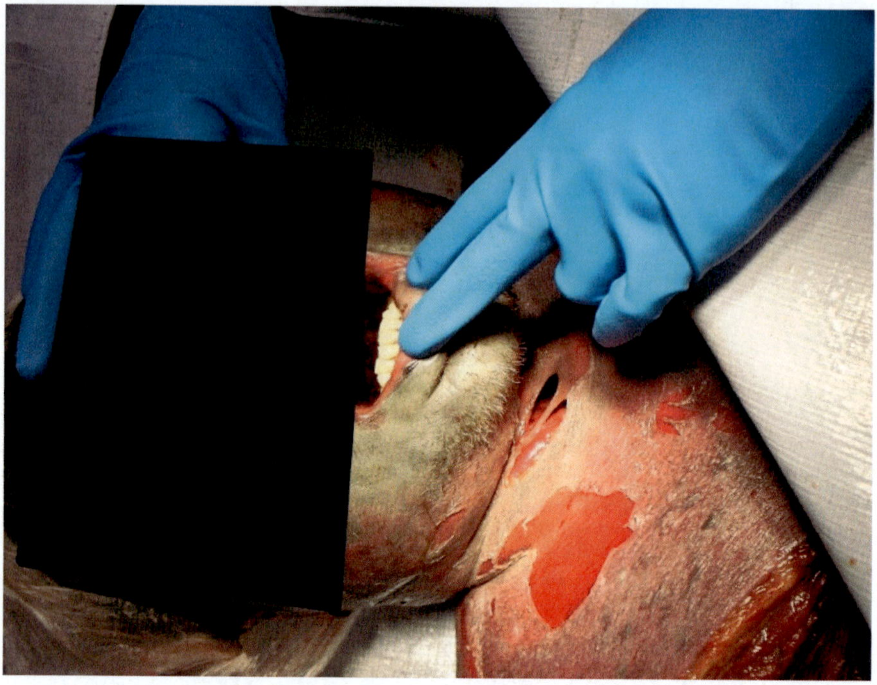

(Photograph of decomposition in water)

One difference will be the types of animals aiding in the biological breakdown of the decedent. Land based decomposition would involve land-based insects, flies, beetles, worms, and the like, in water you will find water insects, crayfish, fish and snails. Water plants also find their way onto and into the decedent. By the time I see the decedent they are in a body bag and are usually post autopsy. Still, I have pulled decedents from the cooler and have found water insects scurrying about in the available fluids. I have also seen an impressive collection of dozens of small tadpoles, some still swimming, in a collection of fluids in the oral cavity. A forensic dentist's goal here is to clean the oral cavity of fluid, debris, and wildlife. I usually accomplish this with a stack of 4" by 4" gauze and a pair of hemostats. I also use cotton tip applicators with long wooden sticks for reach. I know that the oral cavity often fills up again throughout the examination with body fluids. I keep the gauze and applicator tips on hand and touch up as I go.

Depending on the level of decomposition, I take special care not to avulse any teeth inadvertently while performing the postmortem dental examination or cleaning the oral cavity. Most of these water decompositions do not involve having to pry the jaw open to examine them. They are usually loose as rigor is over.

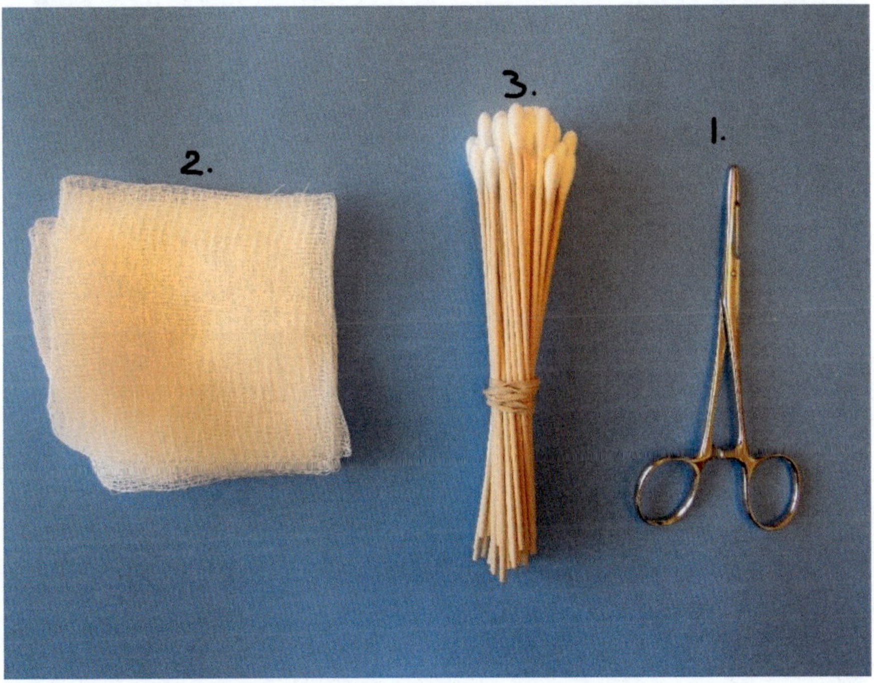

(Photograph of (2) 4"x4" gauze, (1)hemostats, and (3)cotton tip applicators)

Decomposition can also occur on land. Temperature, available exposure to insects and/or animals, time, pH, sun, and rain are a few variables that can affect the speed at which a decedent decomposes. Pictured below is a decedent found in an advanced stage of decomposition with insect activity.

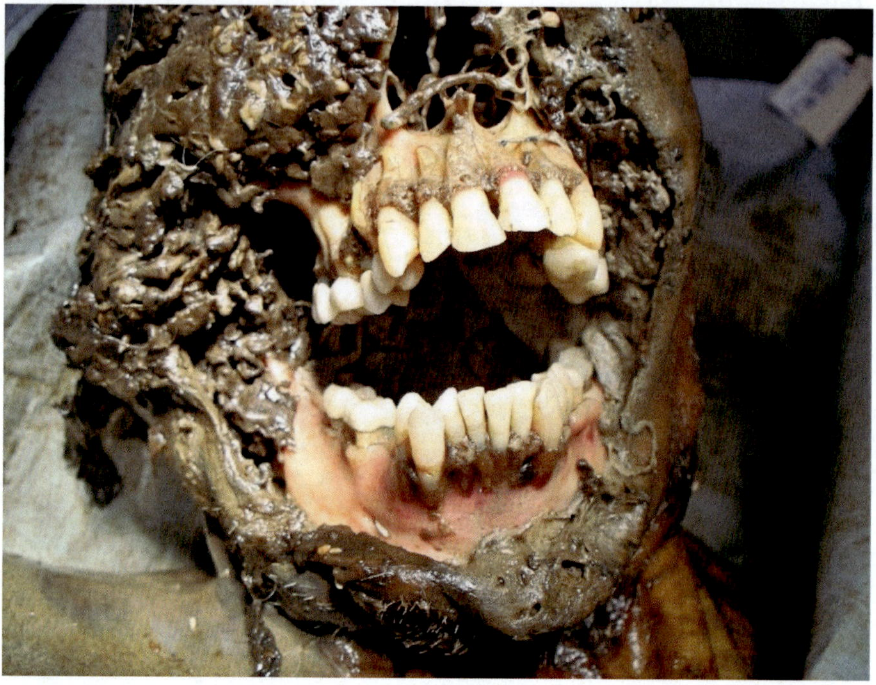

(Photograph of land decomposition with advanced insect activity)

The forensic dentist examining this decedent needs to clean all stages of insect activity from the oral cavity prior to examination. It is too difficult to focus on dental details otherwise.

One lesson I learned from being in the morgue at room temperature is that fly larvae warm up from being in the morgue cooler. They become very active. Some larvae have the ability to contort very quickly like a Mexican jumping bean. They can clear an impressive height. After completing an examination under these circumstances, I realized when I was about to enter my vehicle, that one of these larvae had flung itself into my ear. It sat there quietly and started violently jumping around when I got outside. I try to be more aware of such things now that I got to experience that adventure.

You will also examine decomposition that includes large animal activity. Evidence you need, such as a mandible, can be carried away by a larger carnivore such as a coyote. Teeth may be lost during such feedings. Hopefully enough of the decedent is recovered to make a sound identification. Below is an example of a homicide victim left in the woods with subsequent animal activity.

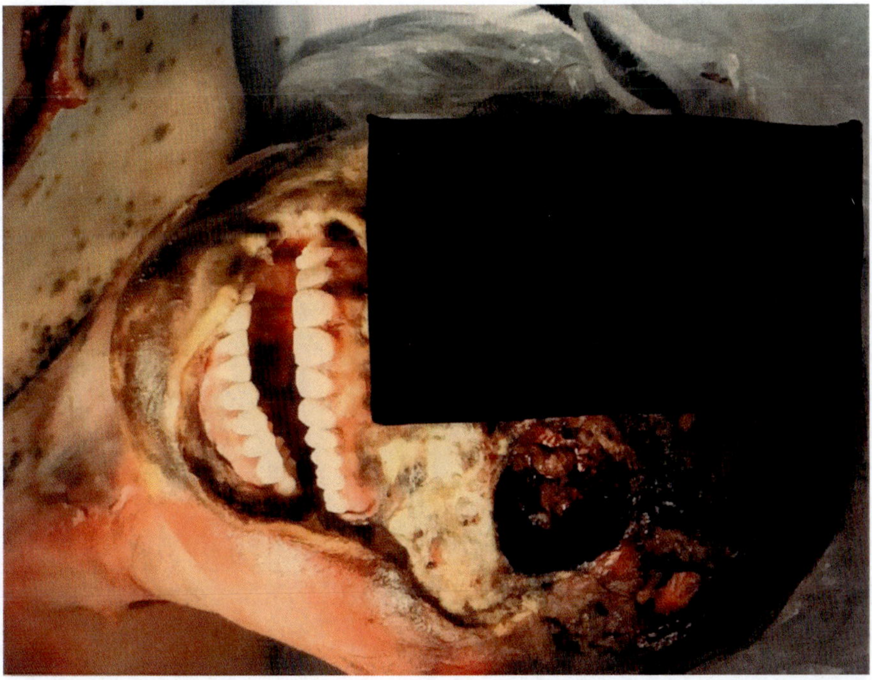

Some decedents are so advanced in their decomposition process they present as mummified, partially skeletonized, or completely skeletonized. Radiographs and photographs are fairly straight forward in these cases. Crime scene investigators may find teeth in the area where the decedent's body is found. The forensic dentist needs to determine if they are human teeth. They can also be tried into the suspected socket where they came from. They can also be radiographed for the future comparison studies.

Below are examples of advanced levels of decomposition on land.

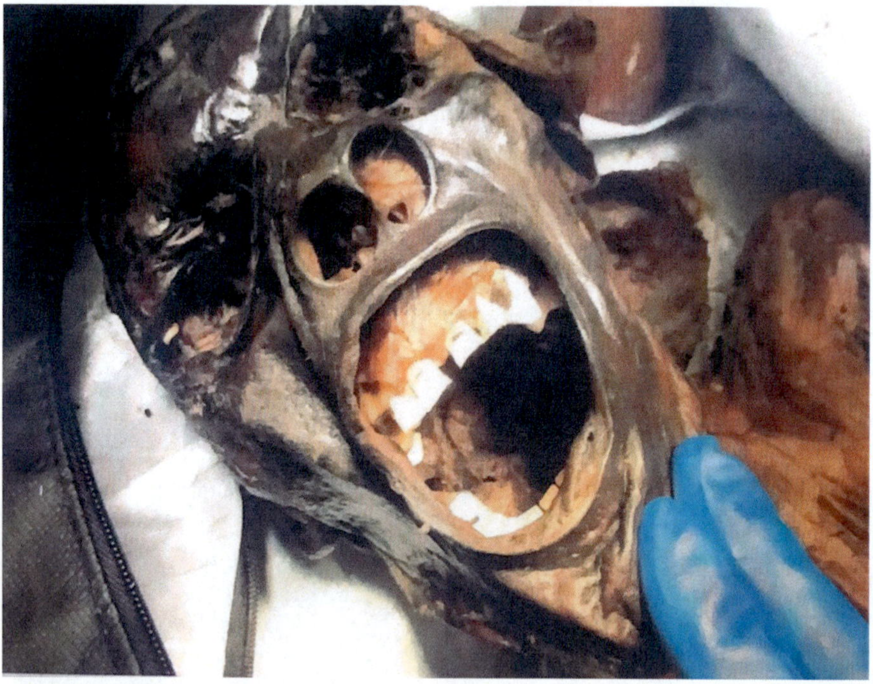

The above photograph displays partial mummification. The skin is dry and leathery. There is little to no moisture left.

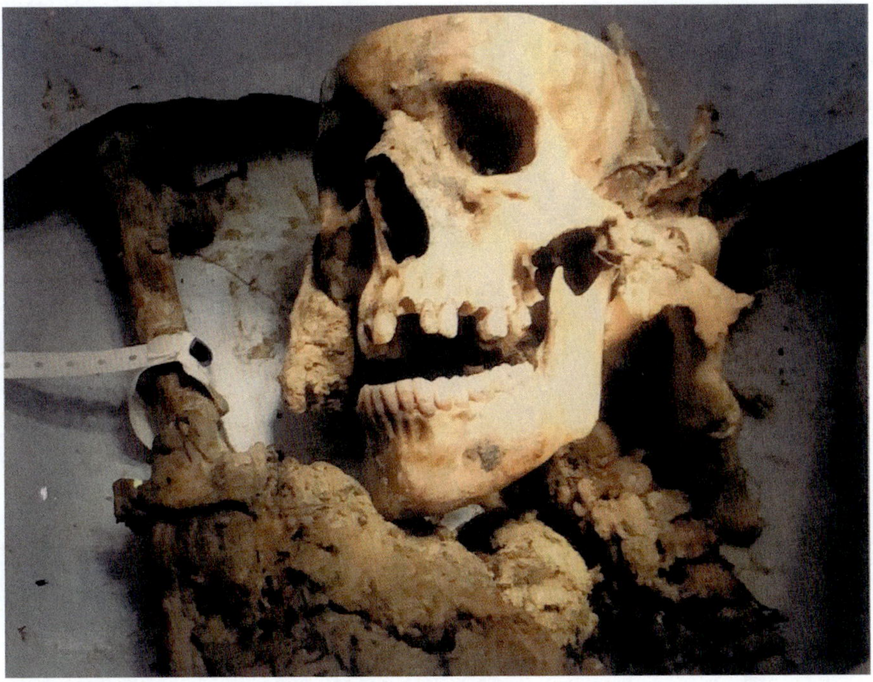

The above photograph is an example of a decedent at the very end stages of the decomposition process.

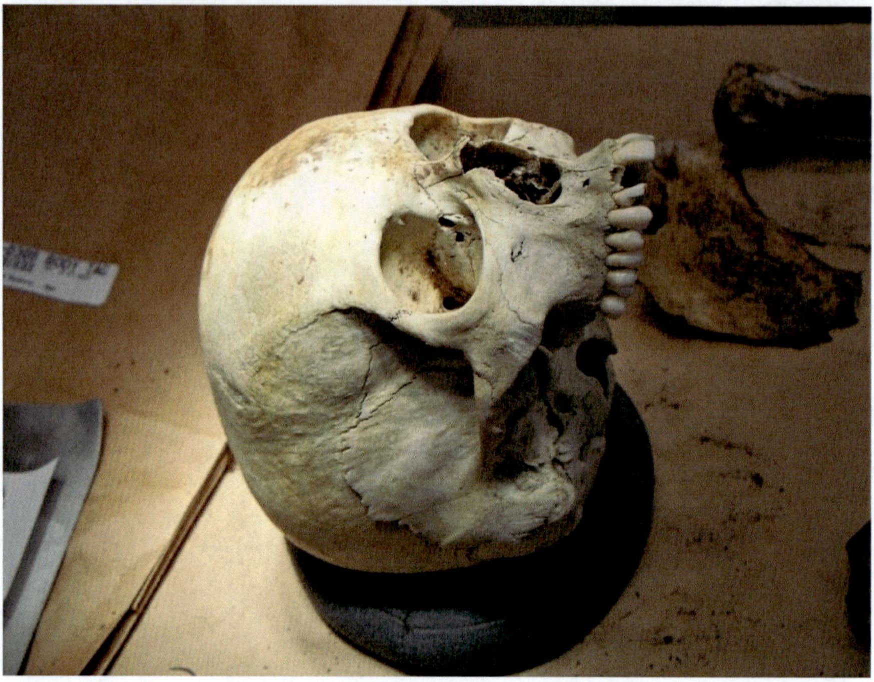

(The above photograph shows only bone remaining after the decedent completed the decomposition process. Radiographs are simple to take here.)

Decomposition will be a frequently observed condition of a decedent for a forensic dentist. Family members cannot be asked to identify a relative in this physical state. Fingerprints are usually obliterated in this stage of death. The forensic dentist can use his skill set to aid in scientific identification, justice, healing and closure can eventually be reached.

Notes Chapter Six

Chapter 7

Chapter VII

Fire

A human body exposed to fire can present a multitude of complications and challenges when performing a postmortem forensic dental examination. Depending on the intensity and duration of exposure special care and extra steps may need to be taken to gather the needed information to be used for comparison studies.

A decedent who had a relatively low exposure to fire can appear quite normal. There may be some minor burning, red areas, blistering of the skin, singed hair and a slight odor related to the fire. In these cases, the examination is mostly straight forward. The teeth are in decent shape. There may be some black discoloration from the smoke and fire. Often times these victims will be viewed via open casket. Special attention must be paid not to assume facial dissection is acceptable. It is here the forensic dentist should ask an investigator if dissection is permitted by the medical examiner. To dissect a victim who is to be viewed makes the work done by the funeral home excessively difficult and can further traumatize a family who is already suffering greatly from a loss. It is by far best to ask for clearance to do any dissection.

Fire victim decedents in some instances can have their mouths carefully pried open enough to successfully clean off the dentition and perform the postmortem forensic dental examination. Below are some of the tools available to accomplish this.

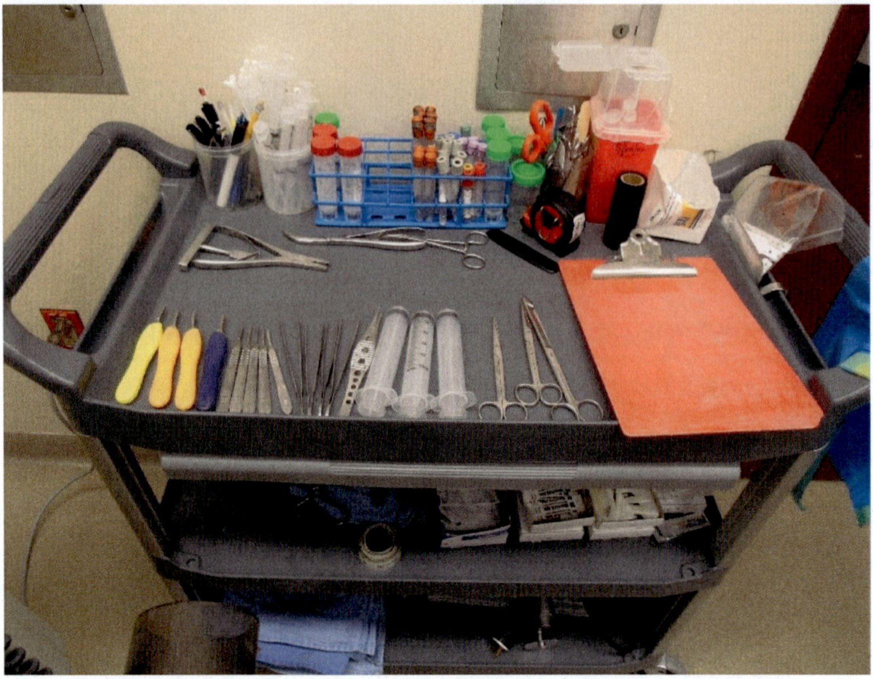

(Photograph of mouth props and pry tools)

The dentist will want to first work the lips open. Next, they will want to place the prying tool between the teeth and gently rotate the tool to see what level of separation can be achieved. The dentist may achieve only a few millimeters up to several millimeters of opening in the anterior region. The dentist must be aware of where forces are placed on teeth. They must try to avoid large restorations as these may fail under excessive pressure The dentist will carefully tease and pry until they can see adequately. Sometimes the facial musculature will relax. This can take time and effort. The dentist may need to prop one side open, examine the opposite side, chart, take x-rays, then remove the prop to repeat the examination on the side that originally had to be propped. Fluids, soot, and debris should be removed as much as possible to afford direct, unencumbered vision. The picture below is an example of a decedent who had minimal external damage due to fire exposure.

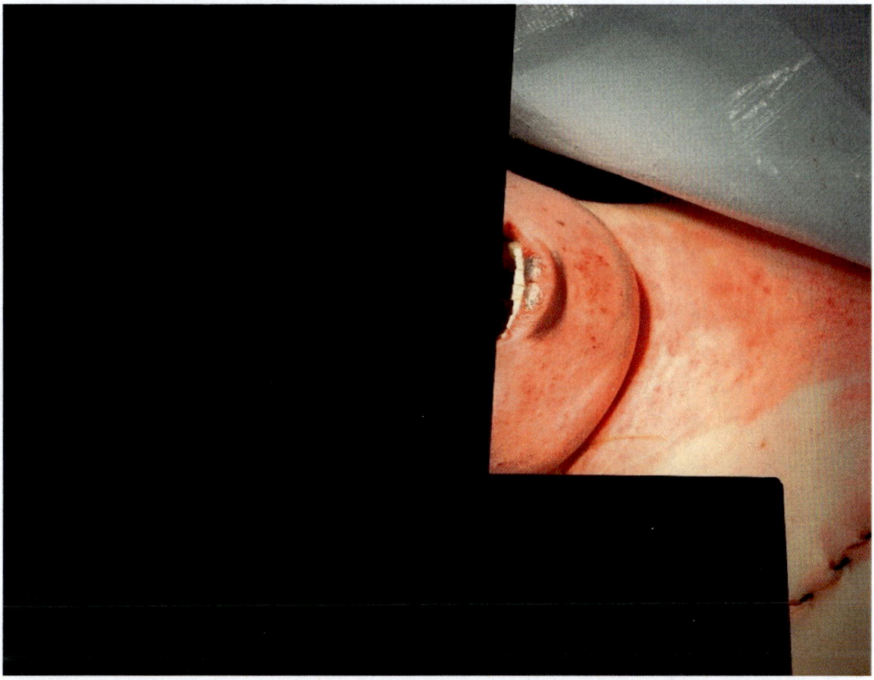

(Photograph of decedent with minimal external damage in a fire)

Taking radiographs may be a challenge. To aid in radiographic imaging, several paper towels can be wadded up in the decedent's mouth. A hemostat can be used to grab the radiograph, place it in the oral cavity, and retrieve the radiograph after it is exposed. Radiographs should be at least wiped off and rinsed before they are bagged for transportation for development. This would relate to the phosphor plates and for chemically developed radiographs. A digital sensor will have its image stored on a laptop. Below is an example of placing a digital radiograph sensor in the decedent's oral cavity using a hemostat with paper towels in place for radiography stability.

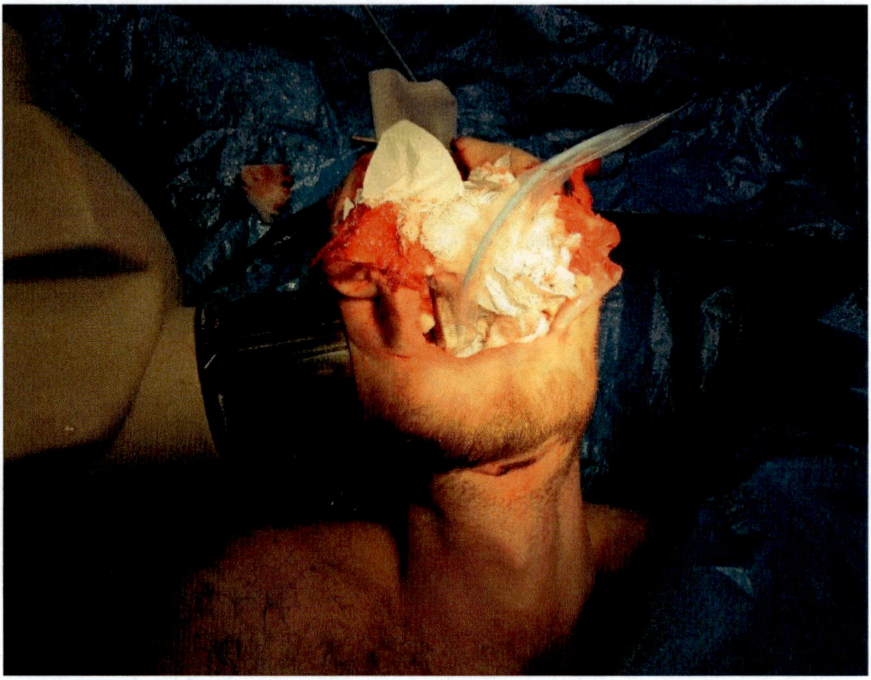

(Photograph of digital sensor being stabilized with paper towels)

Upon completion of the exam, it is appropriate to return the decedent as he/she was found. The head usually has a head prop underneath it. The tools and paper towels used during the examination are removed. The paper towels are placed in hazardous waste and the tools are placed in an appropriate container in the sink. Photographs are taken and the bag is zipped up. At this time, I have a brief, personal, moment of silence with a wish for the decedent to find peace. I do not share out loud what I am doing. It is a personal choice to wish them well and acknowledge their suffering. I appreciate that I get to go home at the end of the examination.

Common courtesy would dictate you pick up after yourself. Also return the decedent to the correct cooler. Roll them feet first and once the decedent is in the cooler they should be feet to the wall as a sign of respect. Thank anyone there that was nice enough to help you at any point in the examination.

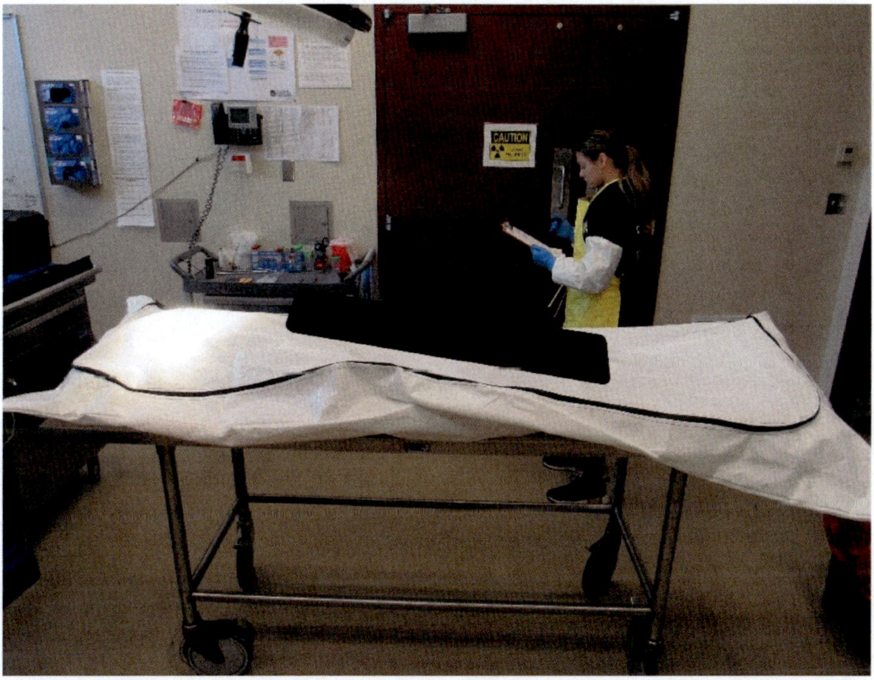

(Photograph of decedent post examination ready for cooler)

There are cases where the decedent has had an extensive exposure to fire, the burning temperature is higher, or both factors are present. In these cases, there is massive damage done to tissue, bones and possibly even teeth. These situations present several areas of concern and special attention.

An extensively burned victim with hardened facial skin and muscle will not be able to have his/her mouth propped open for a postmortem dental examination. This is when the forensic dentist should request permission for facial dissection in order to gather information for comparison and identification. A request to the attending forensic investigator should be made by the forensic dentist to ask the available pathologist/medical examiner for permission to obtain information access by dissection. It should never be assumed by the forensic dentist that you can automatically dissect as you see fit. There may be one or more reasons why this would be unacceptable in this particular case. Dissecting cannot be reversed so clear it first through the proper channels.

Once the forensic dentist has clearance, facial dissection can commence. I personally start at the commissures of the lips with a #12 Bard-Parker scalpel blade and push through until I come into contact with the teeth. I then run the blade through the buccinator muscles, masseter muscles, parotid gland, and various other nerves, fatty tissue, and vessels that are present. If the teeth are tight in occlusion, I will run the tip of the scalpel blade to the teeth in a slow, deliberate up and down motion until I am clean though. If the teeth are not in occlusion, I will run the blade in between the uppers and lowers slowly. The blade does not need to be buried to the handle in this case. It just needs to be through the cheek. If an autopsy was already completed, the tongue will have been removed and visibility is facilitated. If the postmortem dental examination is performed pre-autopsy the tongue will be present. Often the tongue will be found trapped between the upper and lower teeth. It can be bitten down on hard by the decedent due to the fire shrinking the facial muscles during burning. In this case the tongue will be inadvertently dissected by the scalpel. The forensic dentist may try to push the tongue back into the oral cavity although this may be difficult as the bite-down can be severe and the tongue is not pliable at this point. Still, the tongue would need to be cleared away from the dentition to facilitate radiographs and visual examination.

While performing the facial dissection, the forensic dentist needs to pay special attention to any teeth that had prolonged exposure to intense heat. This is particularly important for the upper and lower anterior teeth. This is because as the body burns, the lips and surrounding facial muscles burn, shrink, and retract from the anterior teeth. This exposes the anterior teeth to harsher circumstances. These teeth can become discolored and can be extremely brittle. Just touching them with a finger can cause crumbling. Whatever you can physically see of the anterior teeth should be recorded prior to dissection or postmortem examination. The anterior teeth could be damaged at this point and information lost. Shown below are various stages of severe burning, partial cremation, and dissection steps.

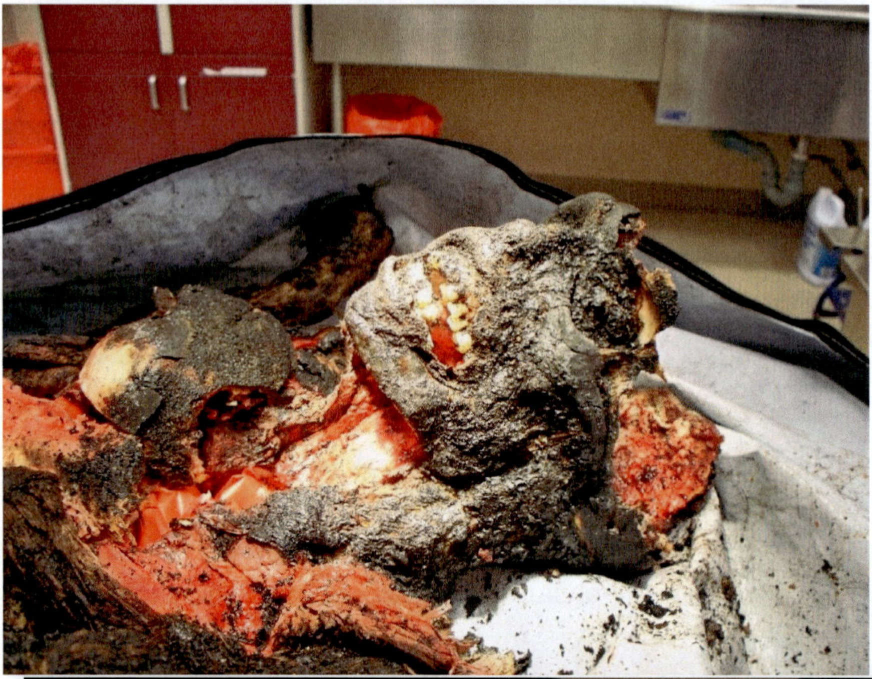

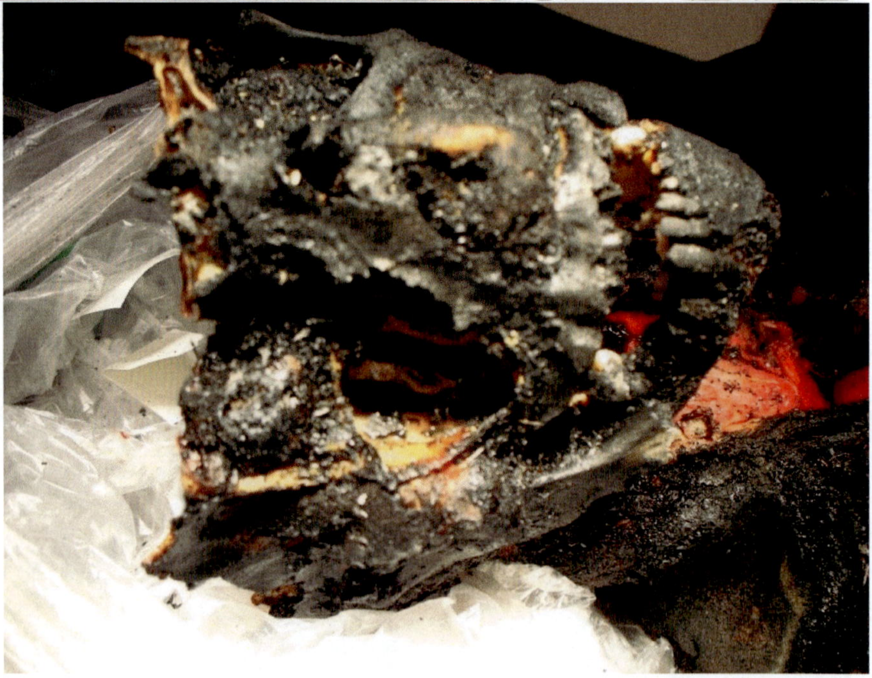

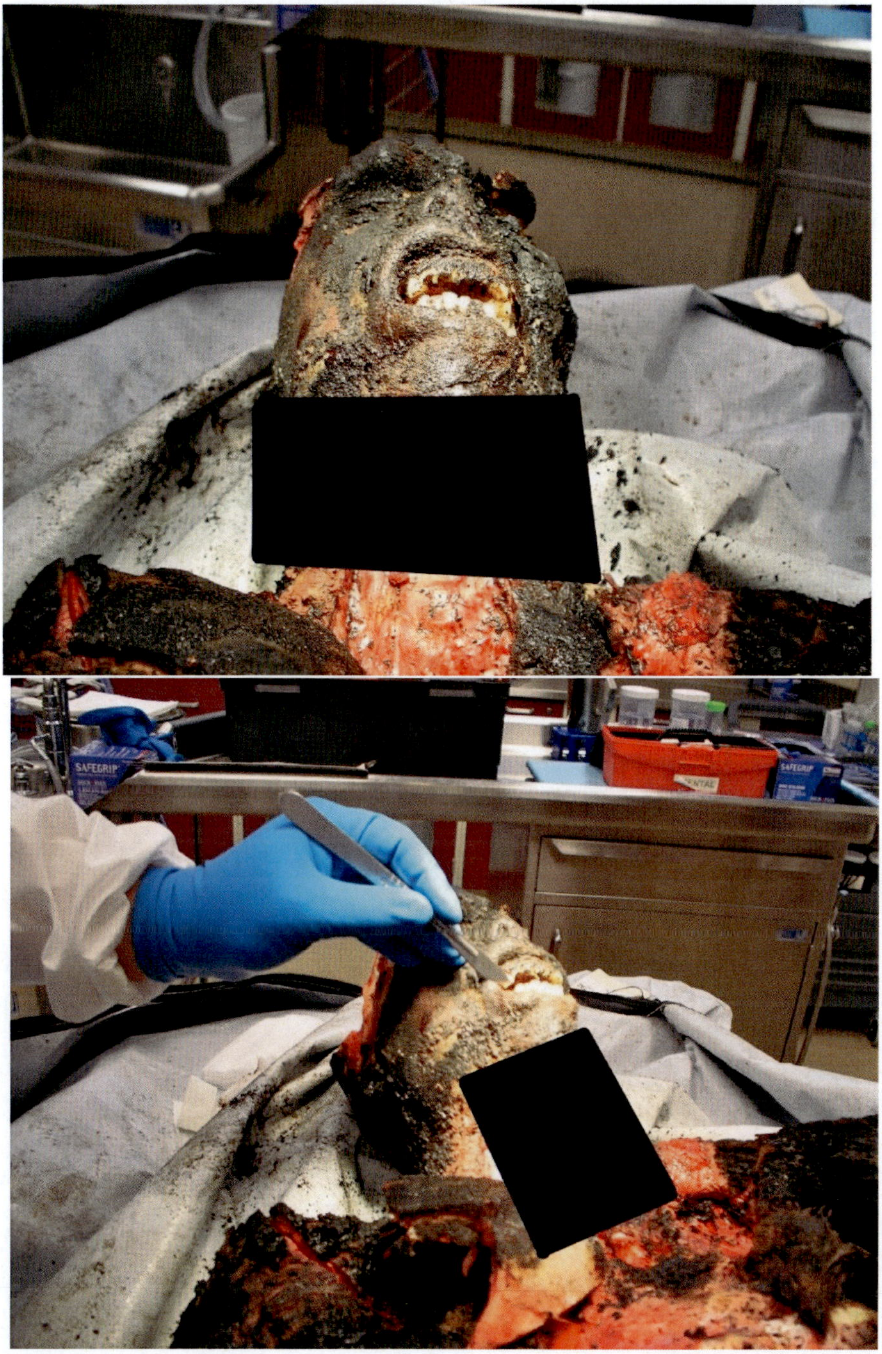

(Photograph of initial incision at the commissure)

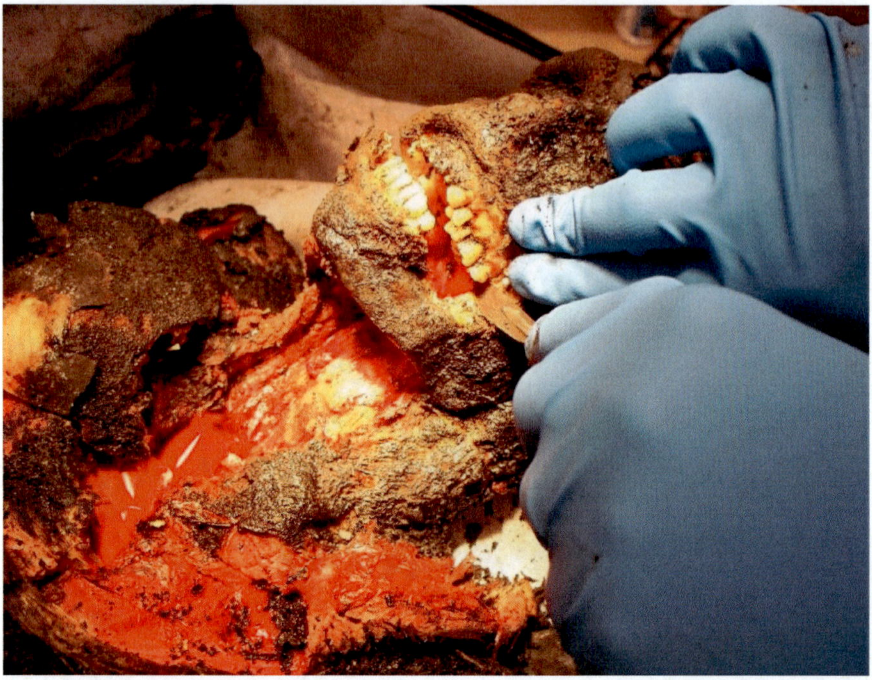

(Photograph of tissue reflection and exposure of dentition)

Once the initial incisions are completed, the tissue adjacent to the upper teeth can be held onto as the scalpel is run along it to reflect the tissue and expose the upper teeth. I choose to start from one side, go across the upper lip to reflect it, then finish on the other side. I then follow a similar pattern on the lower. I do not cut the tissue completely off the face. I leave it attached and only do what is necessary to see what is needed for a satisfactory examination. The molar teeth are usually well preserved from the facial tissues and some pressure can be carefully applied to create space in which to see. The oral cavity will need to be wiped clean to improve visibility. Radiographs can be placed and held steady by using a combination of hemostats and paper towels wadded up inside the mouth to have something for the radiographs to be held against.

These should all be removed and discarded after the examination. The anterior teeth can be charred and very brittle. Some can easily avulse from the sockets as access is being made and the dental examination is being completed. On one hand you need to clean the teeth to examine them. On the other hand, attempting to clean the anterior teeth of severely burned fire victims can destroy them and/or break restorations in them. As a general rule I try to gather as much information on the anterior teeth of severely burned fire victims before I attempt to wipe them off with cotton tip applicators, clean them with gauze or run an explorer over them. Certainly, any prying pressure application to these teeth to open the mouth for viewing will result in broken or destroyed teeth.

Any teeth observed as broken or damaged should be recorded as such. Unless you are positive the break or damage was caused directly or indirectly by the fire simply state the condition of the tooth. For example, tooth #7 may have been charred and broke off during transit. However, tooth #8 was previously broken at the gumline in a fight three months prior, was never repaired, and was subsequently damaged in a house fire postmortem. Just state what you can actually gather from the examination. Avoid hypothetical conclusions.

Once the postmortem forensic dental examination is complete the victim needs to be properly returned to the cooler. Make sure any instruments you used are placed in a plastic tub in the sink. Remove any gauze, cotton tip applicators, or paper towels from the descendant's oral cavity. Radiographs should have been taken and removed from the mouth. Photographs should have been taken by this point. If the head of the victim was wrapped in a plastic bag it should be rewrapped. Any dissected tissue and flaps completed by the forensic dentist during his/her examination should be replaced to its original position.

The body bag can now be zipped up and the victim can respectfully be returned to the cooler.

Notes Chapter Seven

Chapter 8

Chapter VIII

Suicides; Gunshot to the mouth, hanging

Most human beings have an inner drive to keep themselves healthy, productive, and alive. We all work hard for these conditions and even fight for them. Unfortunately, there are people who lose this drive or have never had it. They feel their existence is no longer worth it and they end their own lives.

Reasons for suicide can be many: loss, illness, mental instability, fear of consequence, and lack of hope are a few of the many reasons a person may decide to end their life.

There are many ways to end one's life. Two common types of suicide a forensic dentist can expect to deal with are 1. Gunshot to the mouth and 2. Hanging, the two suicide methods reviewed in this chapter.

A gunshot wound to the mouth suicide case can have a variety of challenges for the forensic dentist based on the positioning of the firearm. These factors can make a large difference in what the forensic dentist needs to do to complete the postmortem forensic dental examination.

A lethal discharge of a firearm above the oral cavity, i.e.) to the temple plays much less of a role in dental identification. The size of the bullet or slug can range from a .22 caliber to a 12 gauge shotgun. As long as the decedent misses the oral cavity the forensic dentist proceeds with their examination in the usual manner.

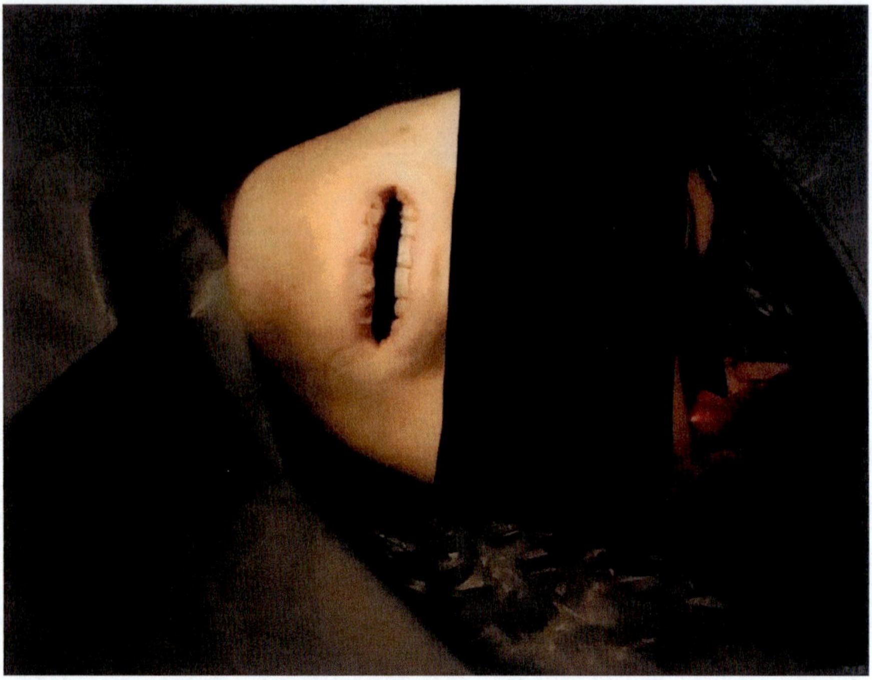

(Photograph of a suicide by a round to the temple (oral cavity intact))

Many suicides are committed by placing the firearm into the oral cavity. This manner of suicide can create a challenge for the forensic dentist. Postmortem dental examination and taking radiographs are no longer straight forward. We will cover some of the challenges created by oral self-inflicted suicide by firearms and what has to be done by the forensic dentist to overcome those challenges.

When a person places a weapon in the mouth it is often in contact with their mandible. When the trigger is pulled the force of the shot pushes the barrel into the mandible and the energy causes fractures with separation. Teeth may avulse (come out).

The mandible can dislocate from the base of the skull. Teeth can also fracture, or pieces may break off. This should be noted when charting future antemortem and postmortem comparison studies. This could help clarify if these conditions were pre-existing or due to the projectile impact.

When taking radiographs, it is best to place the mandible in as close to its original positioning as is reasonably achievable. This will allow easier comparisons to the antemortem records. Often times, strategically placed hemostats and paper towels can aid in this situation. You will have to deal with a variety of twisted tissue, torn muscle, and sharp pieces of splintered bone. These bony pieces can be very sharp and can easily puncture gloves. I find it advantageous to grab things gently at first and slowly apply pressure as opposed to grabbing hold quickly with a lot of pressure while working in a gunshot wound oral cavity. Fractured teeth also can cut like razors. Take your time repositioning the broken pieces and be careful of sharp objects created from the trauma.

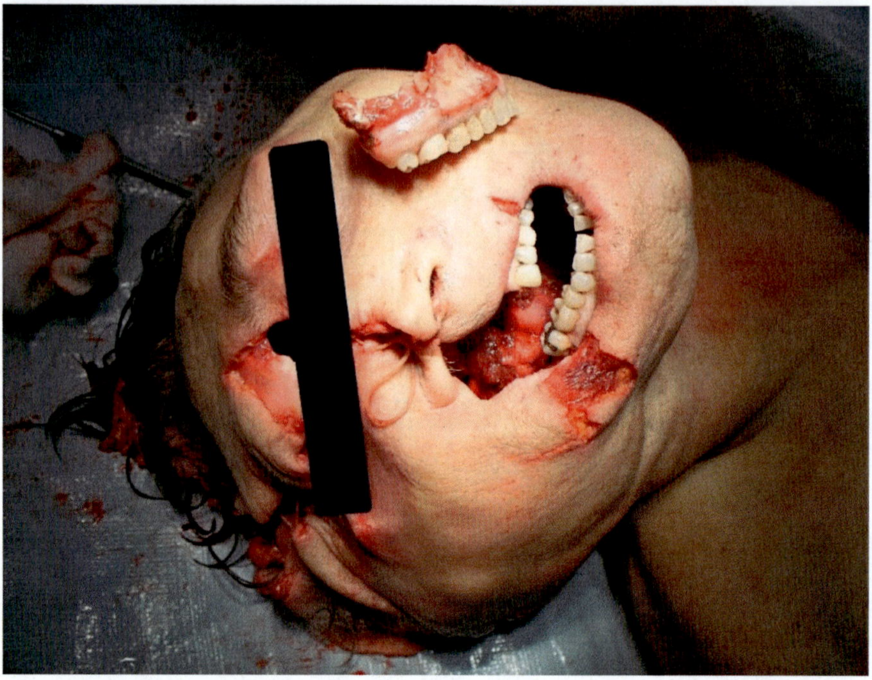

(Photograph of a broken mandible and maxilla due to a self-inflicted gunshot in the oral cavity)

The maxilla usually takes a severe blow from the jarring of the weapon and the projectile fired through the weapon. The tremendous amount of energy that is produced rips open and separates osseous structures, tears through soft tissue, displaces anatomical features, and causes disfiguring trauma.

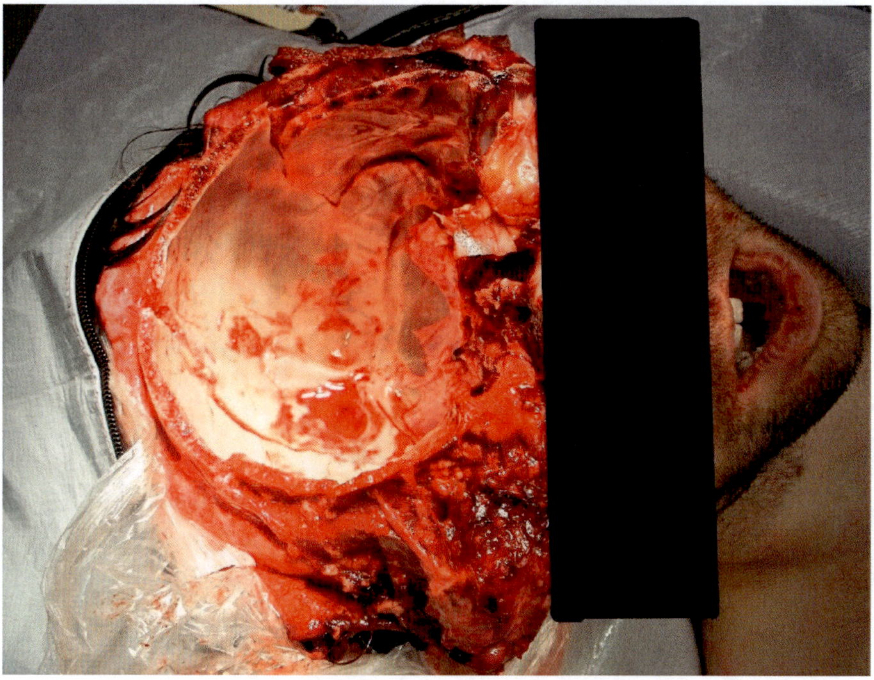

(Photograph of the massive trauma caused by a shotgun through the oral cavity)

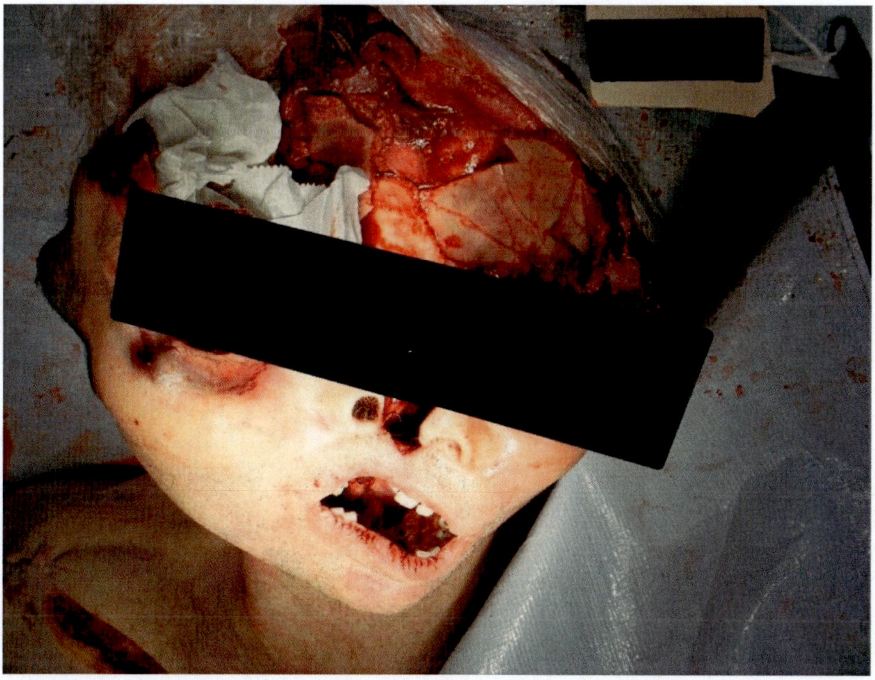

(Photograph of a shotgun suicide through the oral cavity)

Maxillary teeth, like the mandibular teeth, may be avulsed, damaged, or fractured. Sometimes you can replace avulsed teeth in your reconstruction phase. You may also find dislodged restorations that you can "key" back into a tooth for radiographs. The closer you approximate the original condition in your postmortem forensic dental examination the better you will be able to do comparison studies with the antemortem dental charting and radiographs.

Bitewing radiographs are very common radiographs taken in any dental office. If you can manage to approximate the postmortem facial pieces you have from the mandible and maxilla and are able to hold them together to take a reasonable bitewing it could prove very beneficial. This is not always possible but try to accomplish reconstruction as much as is practical. Collect radiographic information to the best of your abilities and as accurately as possible.

In summary, gunshot suicides that involve the wound to the top of the head (i.e., temple) and do not involve trauma to the mouth do not have additional considerations for the postmortem forensic dental examination. In suicides involving a gunshot to the oral cavity, the forensic dentist will have to reconstruct, approximate, and hold in place the mandible and maxilla in order to take radiographs and complete forensic dental charting.

Suicide by hanging generally involves little change in consideration for a forensic dentist to perform the postmortem forensic dental examination. The decedent will generally use some sort of ligature around their neck to break their neck, block airflow, blood flow, or a combination of these fatal situations. Besides a possible mandibular displacement or dislocation, the forensic dentist will usually find the oral cavity and teeth intact and can routinely gather data for his/her postmortem forensic dental examination.

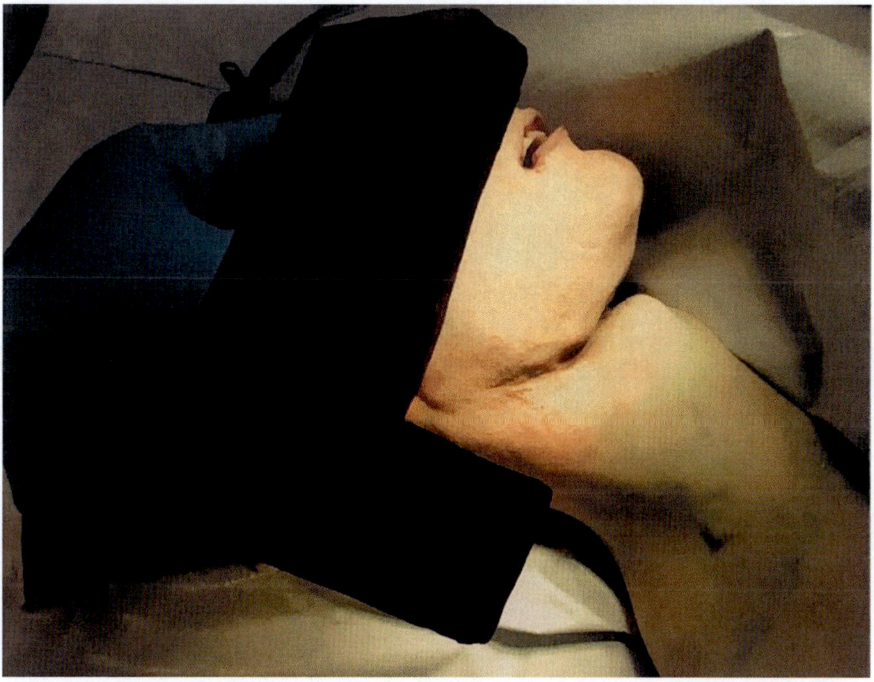

(Photograph of decedent suicide by hanging)

As you can see in the photograph, the damage is done far enough away from the mouth so as to not alter the anatomical features of the oral cavity.

Suicide, by whatever means, is a tragic situation for the person who commits it. The act also has a far-reaching effect on friends and family. Suicides are a common case scenario dealt with by forensic dentists.

Notes Chapter Eight

Chapter 9

Chapter IX

Massive Disfiguring Trauma

There are limitless situations that result in extensive disfiguring trauma of a decedent. Explosions, crushing weight, machinery, high impact collisions, and falling from great heights are a few examples. In these cases, the forensic dentist may be presented with the entire dentition, partial dentition, or pieces of teeth and restorations which may be useful in identifying the decedent. There will be varying amounts of the maxilla and mandible. Some teeth can still be in their sockets within these pieces. Some teeth will need to be approximated in their sockets in order to mimic antemortem conditions.

In this chapter we will be examining 2 decedents that experienced a massive high impact collision. The first decedent was thrown by the collision. The second decedent was dragged and entangled. The third case in this chapter involves skull fragments from skeletonized remains.

The first decedent did not have a firm footing on the ground upon impact. The energy from the striking object was fatal. It threw the decedent into the air and onto the ground resulting in additional trauma from this second impact.

From a dental standpoint this impact did cause fracturing of the maxilla and mandible and disorganization of the dentition.

However, most of the oral cavity was intact. Reconstruction of the oral cavity was manageable. The soft tissue held most aspects of the dentition and supporting bone near the correct positions and to the correct adjacent structures. Through manual manipulation in this case, I was able to rearrange the dentition and supporting structures into a reasonable configuration which approximated the antemortem anatomy. With the aid of hemostats to hold the radiographs and paper towels to hold the shape of the oral cavity I was able to complete the postmortem examination and the radiographs were satisfactory for identification comparison studies with the antemortem radiographs. The key to taking the radiographs in a way to mimic the antemortem positioning is to fill the oral cavity with paper towels. This provides structural support so the forensic dentist can expose radiographs at similar angulations to the antemortem radiographs. This can be a challenging feat considering things tend to shift and slide in the oral cavity when soft tissue is the only binder. Following is a photograph and description of a case with this level of trauma and how placement of paper towels in the oral cavity can aid in providing better postmortem radiographs.

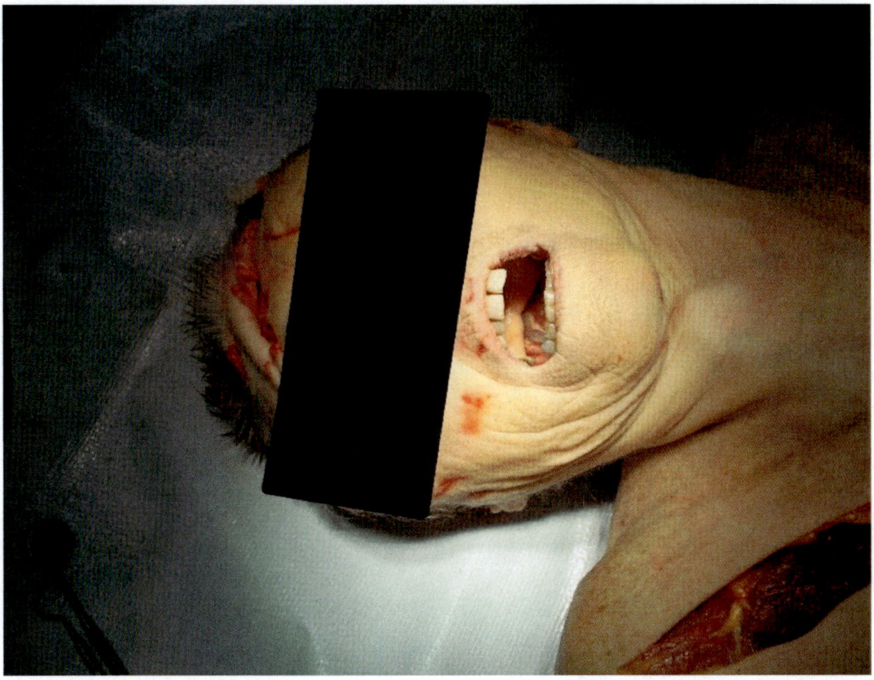

(Photograph of massive trauma with decedent being struck and thrown)

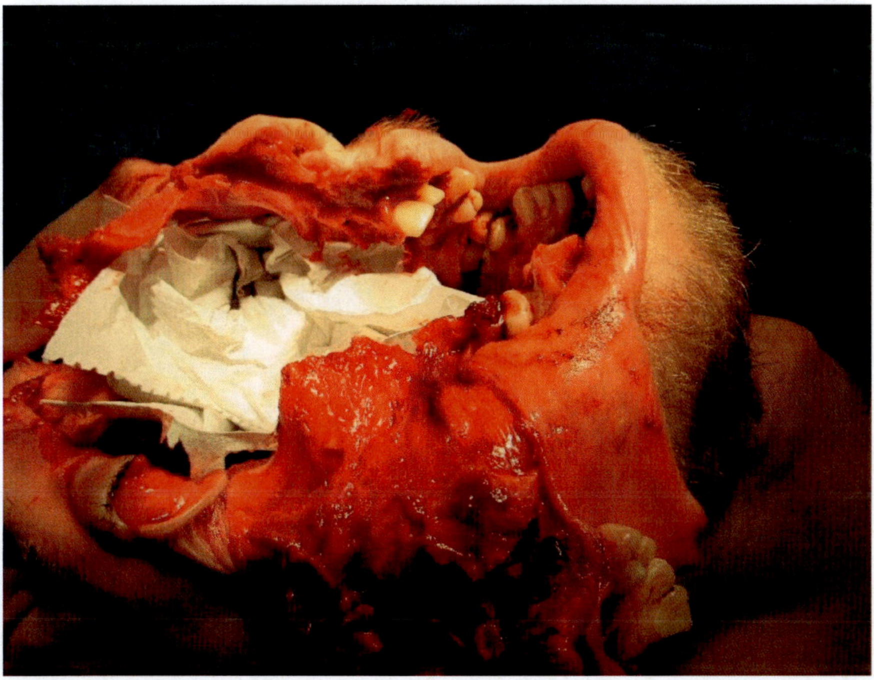

(Photograph of another decedent and how paper towels used in the oral cavity can provide structure to a traumatized oral cavity)

The next decedent example was an individual who was struck by an object of great mass while they had a firm footing. In contrast to being thrown and staying relatively intact as the last decedent, this decedent was struck and torn apart because the striking object had great mass and momentum. The decedent was continually torn apart and crushed over a long distance.

This case was more involved and difficult to reconstruct. Pieces were missing and the collected aspects of the oral cavity were not still connected by soft tissue. The dentition was random and fragmented. Below is a photograph of the condition of the decedent in this case.

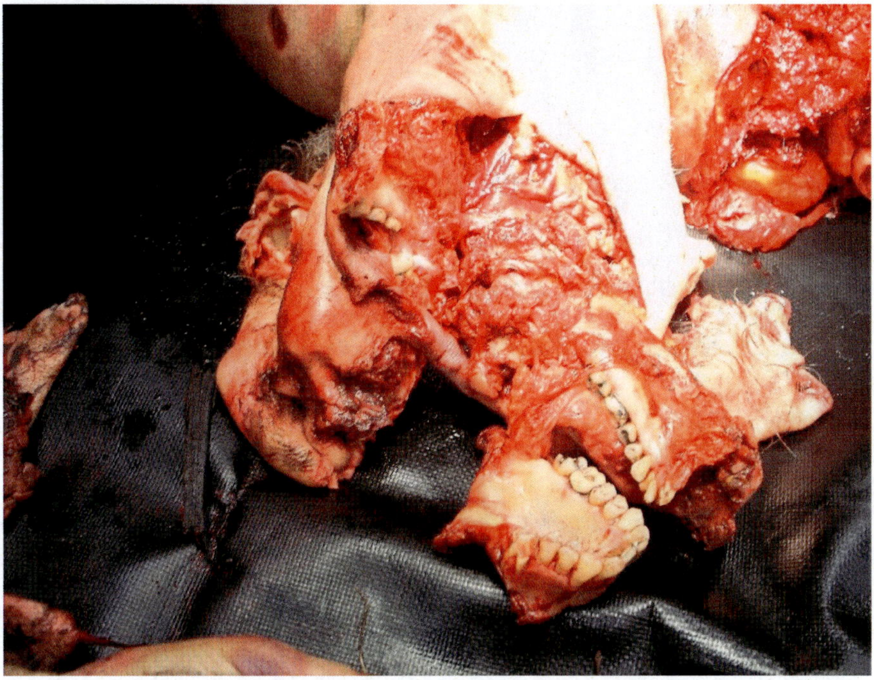

(Photograph of massive trauma with decedent spread over distance)

As you can see it would not be possible to handle this as a routine postmortem forensic dental case. Collecting dentition and parts of the maxilla and mandible and arranging them into a recognizable format needs to be accomplished first. Standard radiograph angles will need to be accomplished piecemeal. The dentist can take comparable radiographs of individual sections of available teeth. They can be lined up "as if" the rest of the oral cavity is present and can result in useful postmortem and antemortem radiographic comparisons.

Sometimes you will be presented with only bone fragments with some dentition. These can be lined up and put together to mimic the antemortem radiographs. Avulsed teeth can be placed back into their sockets. Be careful in this case that there isn't a possibility of there being teeth from another victim. Replacing someone else's teeth into the sockets would negate your comparison studies. Also, the correct teeth need to go into the correct sockets. Take your time with this and if you are not certain you can just radiograph the bone and teeth separately.

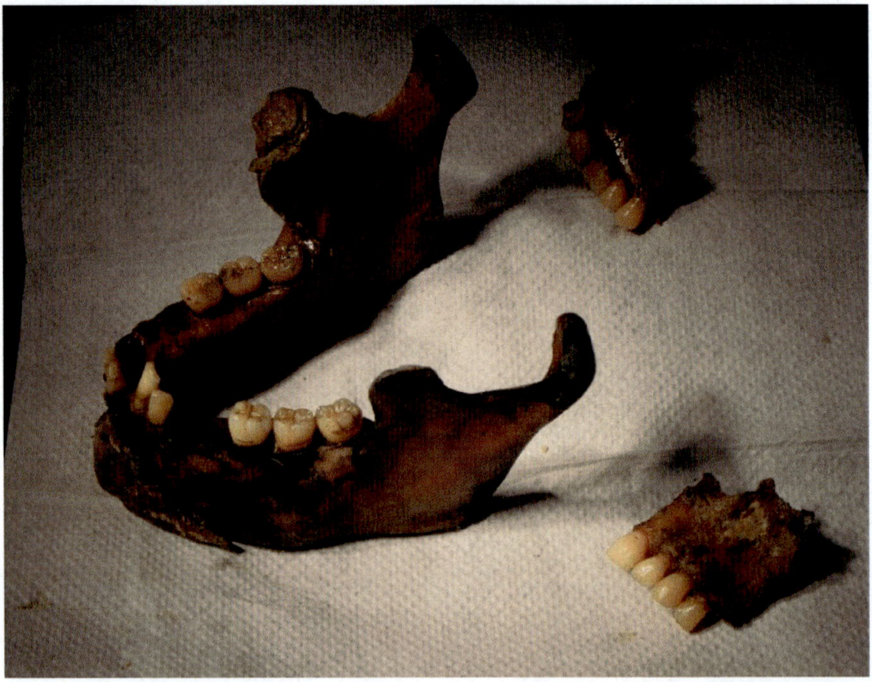

(Photograph of bone fragments with partial dentition)

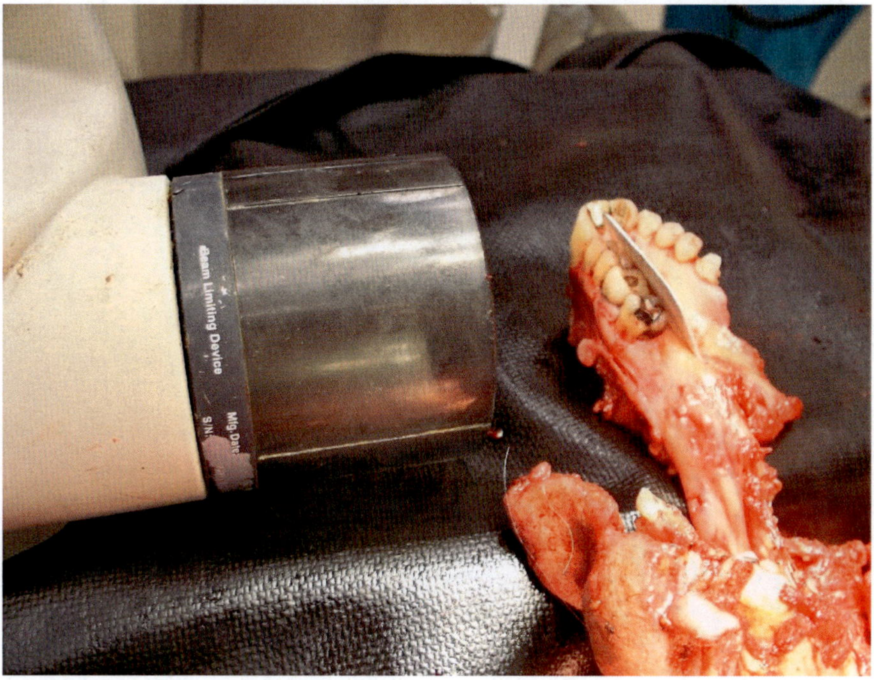

(Photograph of how to take radiograph that would mimic a common position for a bitewing or PA)

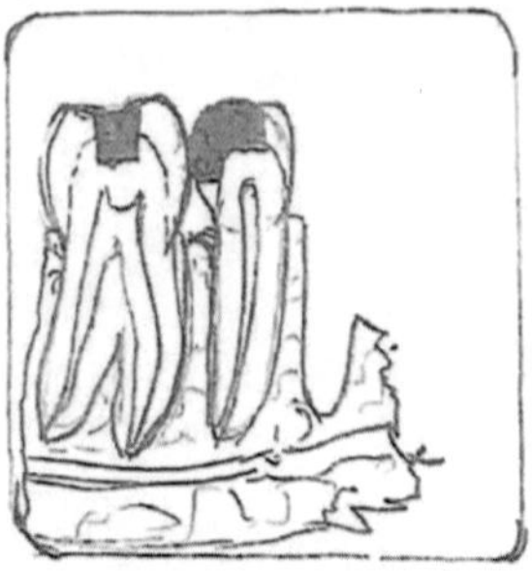

POSTMORTEM

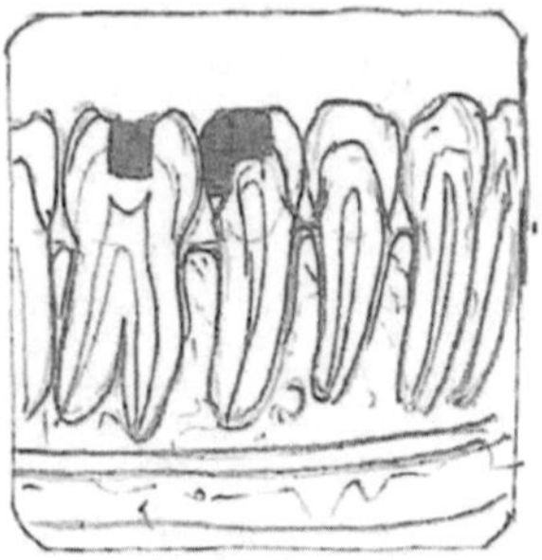

ANTEMORTEM

(Illustration of postmortem and antemortem radiographs when all the anatomy postmortem is not available)

Depending on the condition of the decedent in these and other massive disfiguring trauma cases the forensic dentist will have to overcome challenges to perform their examinations and to take radiographs. There could be a large old amalgam that would be great for comparison that was lost in the traumatic event. The cavity prep in the tooth it fell out of may be used in this instance. There can be a tooth with a root canal, post and core, and crown that had the crown broken off at the gum-line in the traumatic event. In this case the forensic dentist has to look at the remaining root structure, the gutta percha (root canal filler) and the surrounding bone structure. Forensic dentists are aided in their comparison studies since these restorations often have unique shapes and features. When these are lost through trauma or some other event the forensic dentist has to rely on other available anatomical features to do a comparison. It is important to look closely and carefully to make sure every curve to every root matches, every canal is the same shape, every pulp horn looks similar, etc. If they do not appear consistent it is important to figure out why there are differences and if they can be attributed / accounted for logically. For example, a postmortem canal is smaller on a radiograph than the antemortem canal. This could be attributed to the antemortem radiograph being taken when the decedent was much younger. Canals in teeth tend to reduce in size over time.

When you have completed your examination of the decedent you can return the decedent to a (reasonably as is possible) respectful state. Remove any props you may have used and return the decedent to the cooler. Clean the room and put away whatever you used for the examination. You and your assistant should help the investigator clear equipment and return the decedent to the cooler properly.

As the forensic dentist is exposed to more disfiguring traumatic cases, they will learn how to gather the information needed for comparison studies. The dentist will have to think outside their scope of normal education and training in dental school. Experience is an asset. Some questions I like to ask myself when presented with a complicated case are the following:

1. How much postmortem material is available?
2. What shape is the dentition and oral anatomy in?
3. How well can I organize the available material?
4. How can I hold the dentition into position to take useful radiograph?

I then start searching for the answers to my questions. Sometimes there can be a challenge for question #1. A decedent may be presented in a blended, random condition. Teeth and parts of the maxilla and mandible may be found all over within the body bag.

Once you find everything you need you can find answers to questions #2-#4. Breaking the task down into sections can help the forensic dentist complete the task at hand.

If you try to start working on a decedent with massive trauma you can quickly get overwhelmed. If you break your procedures into smaller steps and organize the situation a little bit at a time the task becomes manageable. Reverse engineer the decedent's condition until you can make sense of it and perform your postmortem forensic dental examination properly.

Notes Chapter Nine

Chapter 10

Chapter X

Child Victims, DNA Swabs, Bite Marks

Perhaps the most saddening aspect of forensic dentistry is when the decedent is a child. These are the cases that personally tend to bother me the most. Their innocence and potential in life are tragically cut short. There are accidental and homicidal reasons for their deaths. We will look at examples of both in this chapter. Children tend to explore the world. Unfortunately, they can be injured or killed from their lack of knowledge about what is dangerous to them. They can also be in situations where they are in the wrong place at the wrong time. Car accidents, drownings, and fires may cut a child's life short. We will study an example of a child fire victim in this chapter.

As we have discussed previously in this book, fire victims can be found in a variety of stages of burning. What differentiates a child decedent form an adult decedent as far as a forensic dentist is concerned can be answered via the postmortem forensic dental examination. This example is a young child. Has this child ever been to a dentist? For many young decedents, the answer is no. Even if they had been to a dentist there is a likelihood they did not have radiographs. Perhaps if antemortem dental documentation does exist it may point out some unique features and may provide useful information. Perhaps the records provide nothing, and the postmortem antemortem comparison studies never occur.

The dentist's postmortem dental examination and radiographs are useful in cases where the child is burned too extensively for a relative or friend of the family's to recognize. The examination will allow the forensic dentist to make an age estimation of the child. Although this is not a scientific identification it does increase correlations. This has helped when entire families have been consumed in a house fire. I worked on a house fire with 8 decedents. Four were children. Although no antemortem records were available on any of the children, we were able to assign approximate ages to each child. There our path of identification, correlation, and recognition ceased. From there assumptions had to be made that the 4 unaccounted for children were the ones found in the fire with their positively identified parents. You need to gather as much information as you can as accurately as you can to help progress justice and provide closure. Below: young victim of fire.

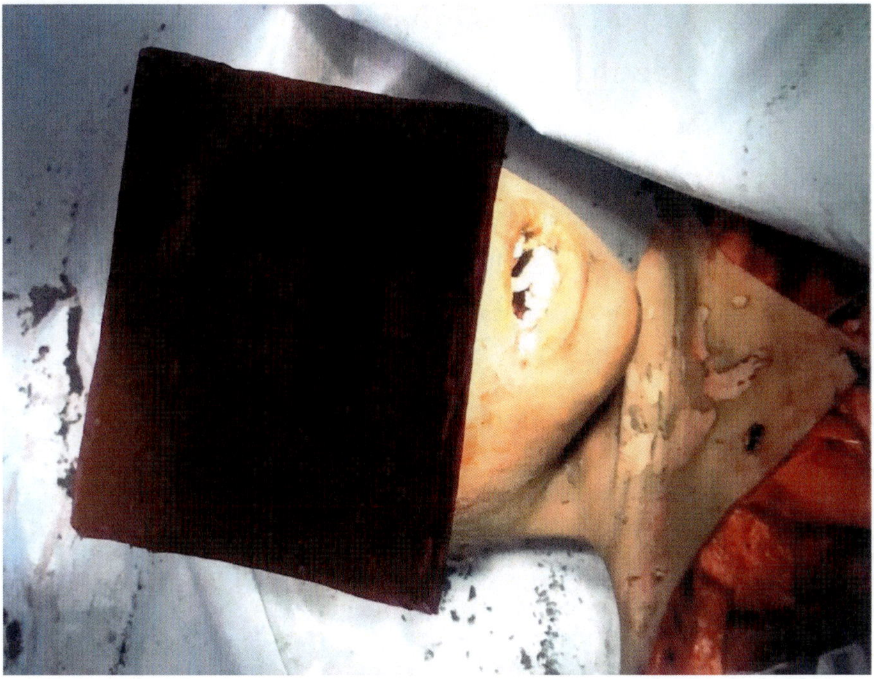

(Photograph of a child fire victim)

Child homicides are perhaps the worst case types you can encounter. I have yet to understand or accept them. There is a need to be respectful of the decedent and their loved ones in any forensic case. Child homicide cases demand the utmost care. I treat the child decedents in any forensic case as if I am dealing with my own child. You need to ask yourself the question, "How would you like your child treated in this situation?"

As we discussed, there may be no comparison due to lack of antemortem dental records. You still want to gather as much information as you can as accurately as possible. At the very least it will provide an age estimation. Look for neglect, untreated large lesions, broken teeth, ripped or torn frenums (tissue attachments between lips and gingiva), cut lips from the inside, and large fracture lines in teeth. These can all be indications of abuse. This information should be relayed to the medical examiner. It could very well bring justice to the child and their family.

Obviously, forensic dentists deal with teeth. Bite marks can also be found on child victims, or any victim of a violent crime. As a forensic dentist you may be called upon to evaluate a bite mark on a decedent. The forensic dentist must know bite mark analysis is not an exact science. Skin is a poor impression material for accuracy and consistency. As a forensic dentist, unless you have specialized training and experience in bite mark analysis, you may do more harm than good by trying to analyze and comment on bite marks. Even for the experts it is a tricky and unpredictable science. It is far less embarrassing to admit your limitations than to overstate what you know. I had one experience with bite mark analysis over a decade ago. I was asked by a prosecutor to be an expert witness in a violent case involving potential human bite marks. I responded honestly. I told him with the lack of experience in bite mark analysis and the uncertainty of bite mark science I would do his case more harm than good. I never heard back from him. This is the correct decision when you are asked to speak as an expert witness when you are not one on that particular subject. State simply what you know and state what you do not know.

When there are bite marks present, a DNA swab can be done to connect the biter to the bite. This is a more accurate method of gathering information than the bite itself. The stakes are high in forensic cases, so the science has to be dependable.

In summary, when the decedent is a child the forensic dentist's role is an important one. There may not be a comparison study done due to lack of antemortem documentation. Even if this is the case a reasonable age estimation can be achieved using the eruption and development patterns of the deciduous teeth and permanent teeth. Bitemarks and DNA swabs can be used by properly trained and experienced forensic dentists to connect a suspect to a case of foul play or to cast doubt on a suspect's involvement in a crime. The forensic dentist has a responsibility to perform within his/her expertise level.

Notes Chapter Ten

Chapter 11

Chapter XI

Is it a human tooth/tooth fragment? Is it an old/ancient decedent?

There are many cases that can be confusing to a forensic dentist. You can feel comfortable when you have an antemortem and postmortem radiograph of an intact molar with a large amalgam restoration that is still situated in the mandible as it should be. Here the forensic dentist can sit back and readily compare the radiographs and the detailed amalgam and determine if the consistencies make for a good argument for an identification.

In the realm of forensic dentistry, we are not always so fortunate. In this chapter we will discuss a complete skull, a tooth, and potential tooth fragments.

A skull was found in a cemetery by a pedestrian, whose dog brought it to his attention. Authorities were called and the skull was brought in for investigation. The skull had a large hole in it; the origins and time of infliction were undetermined at the time of the forensic dental examination. It was an adult skull. There were no existing restorations. Special notation was the level of wear on the teeth. It could be classified as severe attrition. Enamel (in occlusal or incisive contact) was nonexistent.

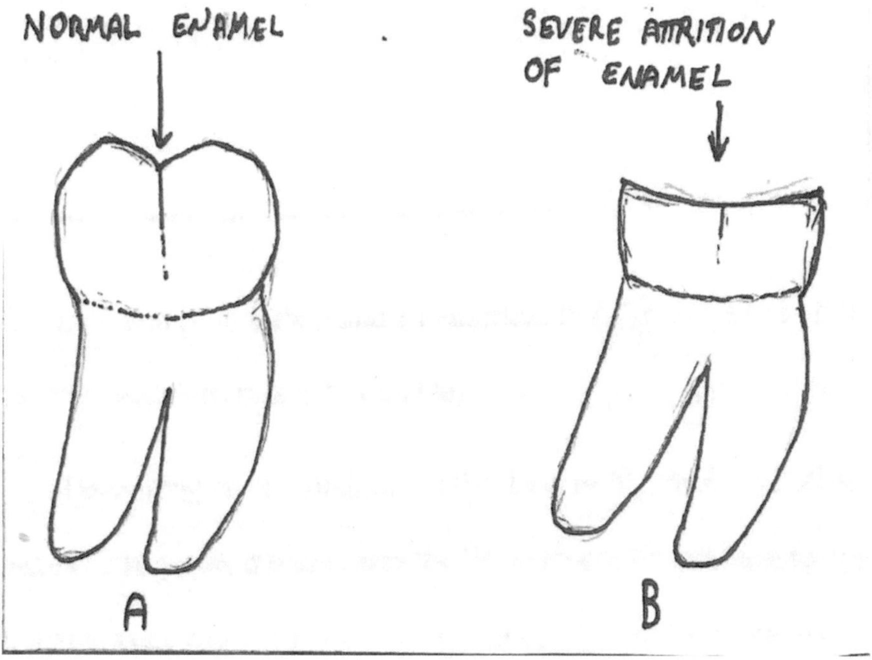

Drawing of: A. normal enamel B. severe attrition

This condition could exist in the United States today. I have not seen wear/attrition to this level in 27 years of private practice. Anything remotely close was accompanied by some attempt at a restoration. There were no potential antemortem comparison records. My conclusion was unidentified decedent. I noted with the lack of any restoration on this adult and the severe wear/attrition on the teeth the decedent could possibly be from previous generations. There were no follow up steps after the postmortem examination.

I could not rule out the decedent was modern. The condition of the teeth and the lack of restorations was atypical for modern times in this region of the United States so the possibility of this skull being from past generations was a consideration. Unfortunately, the postmortem dental examination with radiographs was as far as a forensic dentist could take this case.

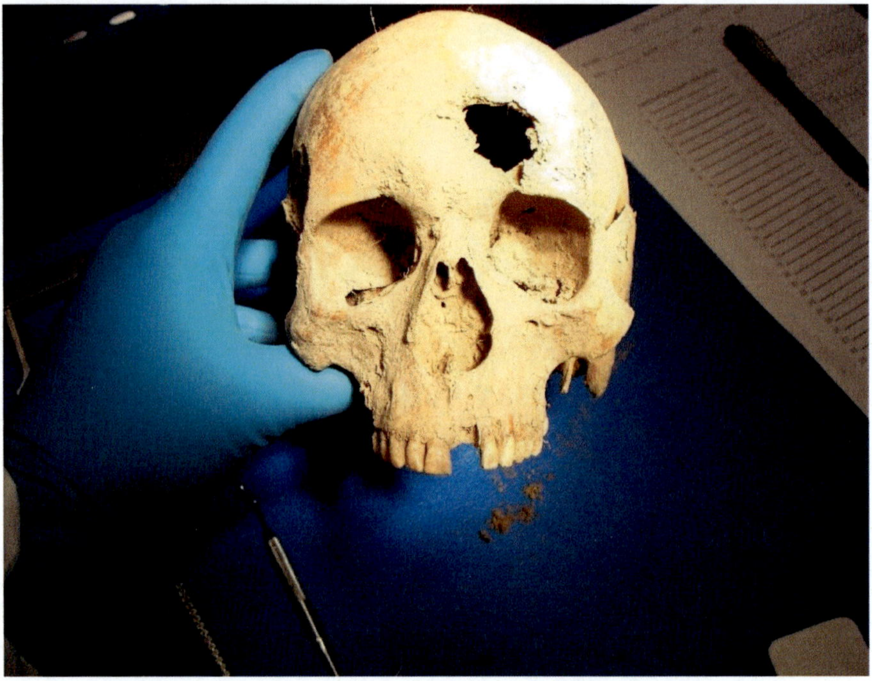

(Photograph of skull found in cemetery)

The next case involved people walking along a rocky beach and coming across a tooth. Concerned, they called the authorities. Examination of the tooth resulted in concluding the tooth was like no other human tooth experienced in my career. It was about the size of a human molar but thinner from a buccal-lingual perspective. It had wear, the cusps were atypical for a human tooth and the roots were bulbous at the apices. The conclusion was the tooth could not be positively identified as human.

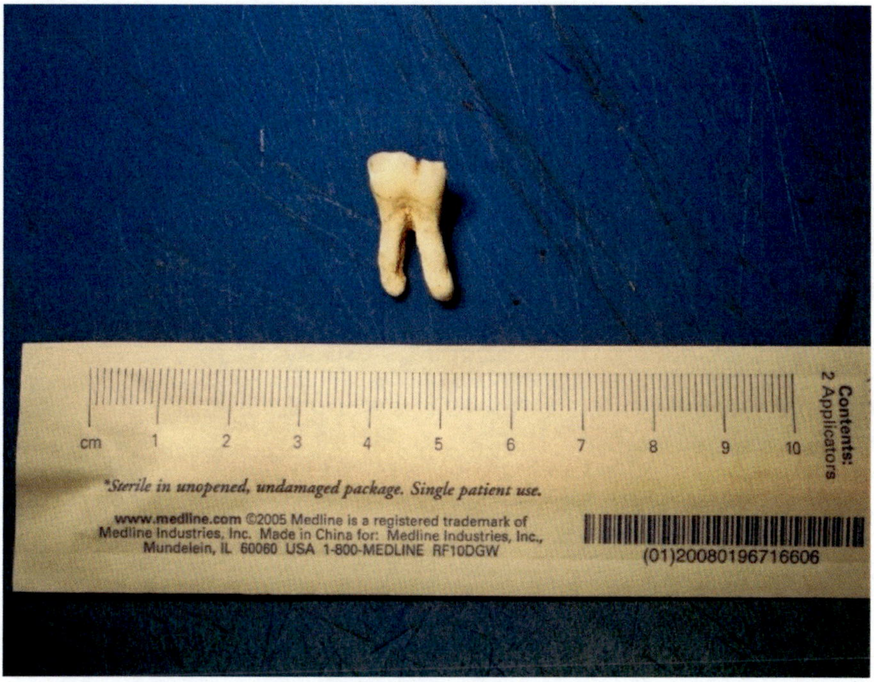

(Photograph of a tooth found at a beach)

Another suspected human tooth was found while digging near an old house. Authorities were called. Forensic dental examination showed a tooth appearing much larger than a typical human molar. Although anatomical anomalies do occur, it was unlikely this tooth was of human origin.

In both of these cases subsequent DNA testing may have provided more insight as to the actual origins of these teeth. After completion of the forensic dental examinations, the forensic dentist is finished with the case.

In another case, this one a homicide, several fragments, possibly of teeth, were found on scene. A postmortem forensic dental examination was performed. I used magnification to better evaluate detail. Most of the pieces were too porous to be dentin or cementum. Small canals could also be observed. This is not observed in enamel, dentin, nor cementum tooth structures. The piece to the naked eye did indeed, very much so, look similar to crushed and damaged tooth structure. I had to rely on magnification to find clues pointing toward them not being dental in origin.

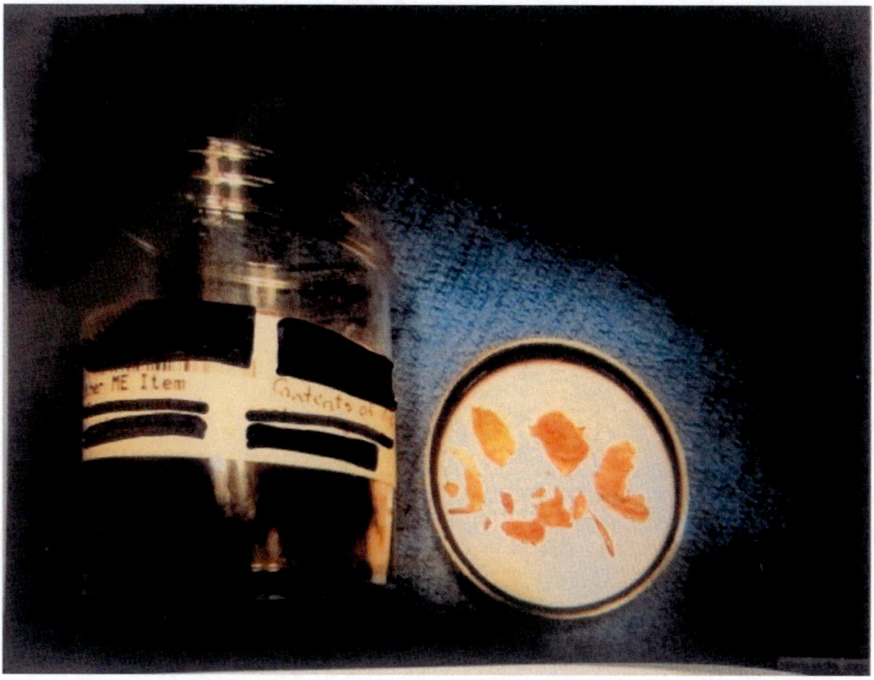

(Photograph of suspected tooth fragments)

It is great for a forensic dentist to be presented with a case where the teeth of the decedent are intact, heavily restored, have unique features, and are accompanied by excellent antemortem charting and radiographs. Here, comparisons can be made relatively easily, and conclusions can be drawn. It is when the forensic dentist receives less than perfect teeth, fragments or nearly destroyed decedents that he/she really needs to double down. As disappointing as it can be, there are cases where you will do a complete and through postmortem dental examination and make no conclusion as to the identification of the decedent or even if it was a human decedent. The urge to overreach to draw unsubstantiated conclusions must be fought. Intent to help can have the opposite effect. Sometimes you can only go so far in an investigation. This in itself is useful and should not be written off as a “waste of time.” It is a science and scientific methodology should be followed. It strengthens the credibility of the forensic sciences by not having an answer to every question.

Notes Chapter Eleven

Chapter 12

Chapter XII
Court

A Forensic Dentist can be expected to discuss his/her expert conclusions in a court of law and be cross examined. The identity of the decedent, obtained scientifically, can and does play a significant role in court. Imagine what would happen in a Homicide trial if the Defense Attorney asked the prosecution what scientific evidence they have that the victim is who they are claiming it to be. What would happen if the prosecution responded "Well…we think that the victim is…"? You logically cannot expect a jury to take away a defendant's freedom, possibly for the rest of their life, when the prosecution is guessing the identity of the victim.

A Forensic dentist doesn't use the science of DNA recognition. They don't use fingerprint data bases or rely on a friend or family member to confirm identity.

The forensic dentist gathers radiographs, photographs, and clinical examination data postmortem. He/She then, when available, compares these findings to antemortem radiographs, progress notes, photographs, and charting. Consistencies are recorded and identification conclusions are reached.

After the comparison is complete and written up with an investigator's signature, the forensic dentist could receive a subpoena to appear in court to provide expert testimony. The steps involved can vary from case to case and from district to district. I will review my personal experience in my first court appearance.

I completed a postmortem dental examination on a homicide victim two years before I was subpoenaed. I took several radiographs and photographs as there were several upper and lower teeth remaining. I charted and documented the decedent as usual.

Later in the week I received a call from the morgue that the antemortem radiographs and charting were available for review. I headed downtown after my regular workday at my dental office. When I was presented with the antemortem dental records I was disappointed to see there was only one radiograph of less than optimum quality. It was, however, readable. It was taken in order to remove a tooth root which was obviously not there for comparison in the postmortem radiographs. The antemortem records did state that the root was removed and that made situational sense. Luckily two more teeth were on the antemortem radiograph. They had unique characteristics such as root canal morphology, rotation, attrition, and bone support levels. These were studied and compared for some time. The features were all radiographically consistent. The findings were written, but not overstated, on the provided dental identification sheet. I had taken a radiograph that was in nearly the same position as the antemortem radiograph. The other postmortem radiographs were not useful in the identification process. Since one should not review radiographs or charting prior to one's postmortem examination one will usually have extra radiographs. You can do a successful identification with one tooth, but you need its image on both the antemortem and postmortem radiographs to be successful. If an investigator tells you only bitewings are available antemortem, make sure you take postmortem bitewings but do not review the antemortem bitewings prior to your postmortem examination.

I heard nothing further about this case for several months. One day at the office a subpoena from the district attorney's office showed up. As per my usual character flaw of paranoia I wondered "who the hell is coming after me?!" I opened the letter to find I was to appear in court by order of the prosecution to provide expert testimony as to how I came to the conclusion the victim is "Victim X."

This was my first time testifying as an expert witness. This was the first time I sat in a courtroom except for a speeding ticket in college. I felt I did a good job in the identification process but had no idea what to expect.

Fortunately, I had a briefing and mock questioning session from a helpful Assistant District Attorney who would be asking me questions on the stand. I also benefitted greatly from coaching from two friends. They were a court experienced forensic pathologist and a law professor.

My friends reassured me and told me to remember that I will be the only dental odontologist expert witness in the court. They encouraged me to answer questions with simple answers and not to elaborate. They also said if there were any questions that were misleading or were framed in such a manner that they cannot be answered without clarity, address the defense, and tell them you did not understand the questions as it was asked, or you can't answer the question as it was asked. They both warned me to watch for traps by the defense to discredit me.

The ADA reviewed questions that were straight forward and required short answers. Questions like "Who do you work for?" "How many years have you been working for x?" and "How many forensic ID cases have you completed?"

By the time these conversations were completed I felt more confident in what was to transpire. There were over seventy witnesses to be called on this case and I was one of the last to go. This is how trial went for me.

I went through security and was checked for weapons. I was brought hurriedly through several hallways and doorways to the outside of the courtroom by someone from the DA's office. Things moved quickly. As I got to the outside of the courtroom, I was told I will be on fast so be ready. Within a minute a Sheriff's Deputy opened the door, looked at me, and said "Dr. Winkler? Go to your left, go to the front by the judge, stop there, and get sworn in."

I did as I was directed. I walked past the observers, jurors, ADA, defendant, Defense Attorney, Stenographer, and stopped to be sworn in. The judge welcomed me in and told me to have a seat. There was a microphone there which I spoke into way too loudly. After that I quickly adjusted my volume.

The ADA asked similar questions as in the practice run. Name, how I became a Forensic Dentist, how identifications are done. The one question she did ask that was not reviewed was the name of the victim as determined by the forensic dental exam! It had been more than 2 years since I completed the case. I do not know the names of the decedents (around two hundred) that I have examined. Fortunately, I studied the case earlier that morning and I stated the name after an awkward pause. The ADA thanked me said no further questions. I thought this was great and was ready to get excused. Before the trial, the ADA said she couldn't imagine me getting cross examined by the defense because she figured the defense would not want the jury to hear my testimony for too long because it could be considered graphic and work against them.

Surprisingly, the Defense Attorney stood up right away. He asked if I had been to dental school in Buffalo. He tried to make a connection to me by asking if I knew a certain person. The ADA objected. A few more attempts to trip me up were as follows...

Defense ATTY: So, when you take an x-ray, you know how to orient it by looking at the antemortem films?

Me: No. As I stated, I do not review antemortem films prior to my postmortem examination.

Defense ATTY: So how did you take a similar x-ray?

Me: I took several. One was similar enough to compare.

Defense ATTY: So, you use the antemortem x-rays you take so how do you tell from one film...

Me: I don't take antemortem films. When I see the decedents, I can only take postmortem films. (I cut him off...)

Defense ATTY: Of course. How can you tell from only two teeth who a person is?

Me: You can look at the angels of alveolar bone recession, root morphology, root canal morphology, attrition patterns constrictions and shapes and abrasions at the cemento enamel junctions, rotations...

Defense ATTY: No further questions. Thank you, Dr. Winkler. (He cut me off...)

I may have gotten a little too technical for the Defense Attorney. I saw his eyes get big and his mouth opened up a little. He shuffled some papers on his desk and said he was done. I may have missed a word or two but that is fundamentally how the cross examination progressed.

When the Defense Attorney finished his questioning the judge paused, looked around the courtroom, and then looked at me.

"Thank you, Dr. Winkler, you are dismissed." This trial was during mask mandates. I was required to wear a visor and sit sideways to speak into the microphone so the courtroom could hear my testimony. I thanked the judge and quickly exited the chair. I forgot the microphone was stuck under the facial visor so when I stood up there was a horrific, loud screeching, banging noise. The entire courtroom jumped. I grabbed the microphone; said I was sorry and took off at a fast pace from the courtroom. I had the pleasure of walking past everyone I just scared with the loud noises I made.

Less than one week after I testified, I was told the verdict. The defendant was found guilty and given 25 years to life. I was told the jury was heavily persuaded by the Pathologist, the Forensic Investigator, and the Forensic Dentist. It was definitely a team effort, and it was gratifying to play a role in justice being served.

I had some take home lessons from being an expert witness in a homicide case.

1. Look at and complete every case you do as if it will be questioned and analyzed in a court of law.
2. Do not talk too much or overstate the answer to a question.
3. Do not overstate your abilities.
4. Pay attention to details. Be specific with your descriptions.

5. Review your case before you take the stand. Make sure everything is fresh in your mind including the victim's name. The ADA and I did not review knowing the victim's name. I knew a case number. Luckily, I read an article on the case earlier in the day and the victim's name was in it. This would have been awkward had I not known.
6. If during cross examination the Defense Attorney is framing you with his/her questions so you cannot answer without sounding like you are unsure of yourself or contradicting yourself, do not try to answer him/her. Ask the Defense Attorney to restate the question due to it being ambiguous as it was asked.
7. You are the expert witness in the room. You are the one who knows what is truthful to say and know what isn't truthful to say. Do not compromise what you know as truth.
8. If it beneficial to do research before you go court. Connect with experienced people. A ten-minute discussion with them can prove extremely helpful in the way you are viewed by the jury, the judge, the defense, and the prosecution.

Notes Chapter Twelve

Conclusion

Conclusion

This book contained several examples of what a forensic dentist can expect to see when called to a case. It is not all inclusive. In general, a forensic dentist should remain humble and respectful. He/she should also be attentive, look for details, and document the case well. State what you see clearly while avoiding jumping to conclusions when the science or evidence is not there to support it.

Try to be as helpful as possible to the investigators, security guards, techs, police, and pathologist as you can. Your contribution and time spent on the case should be welcomed by all because you are a good team player who's small but significant role in the case includes a healthy attitude and a positive drive which boosts the people you are working with. Remember the people you share the case with are surrounded by death and misery on a daily basis. If you are doing forensic cases on a part time (as needed) basis you can and should put in the effort to make others feel happy about you working with them as a forensic dentist. Recognize when you are being helped. "Thank you" and "I appreciate you helping me" are terms that are underutilized but cannot be overutilized. Have pride in your work. Know you are helping others and enjoy the learning process when it presents itself. Forensic Dentists are very few in number. Know your importance and take the opportunity to better the people you work with.

As you progress through your forensic endeavors you also may want to think about how to protect your information. The material you are involved with is not something intended for public viewing. I recommend not taking any forensic photographs on your cell phone. Anything downloaded onto your computer is also hackable. I had my intel hacked into by hostile forces when I was a military officer. They infiltrated thousands of military officers and their families. This was secure in the Department of Defense. I am sure if that can be breached your laptop or phone can be. I keep my cases and photographs offline, so I do not have to worry about being compromised.

If you are not a forensic dentist and don't plan to be one, my hope is that you now have a decent understanding of how forensic dentistry works and how it relates to the other parts of the forensic team. We all utilize scientific methods to gather and interpret each case. We all benefit by reporting truthfully, accurately and without arrogance. We are dealing with the end of a fellow human's lifespan here on Earth, a lifespan that has been tragically cut short by suffering and death. By sharing my real life experience with you, I hope you have a better grasp of what needs to be accomplished forensically when a decedent of any condition is discovered under these tragic circumstances. Thank you for your interest! I hope you continue to learn forensic methodology as I plan to and better yourself with time.

Notes Conclusion

Made in United States
Orlando, FL
04 November 2026

90202068R00083